Silvina Gendler

Prevalence of Transfusion-Transmitted Infections

Silvina Gendler

Prevalence of Transfusion-Transmitted Infections

In donors of an Intrahospital Blood Bank of the Autonomous City of Buenos Aires

ScienciaScripts

Cover image: www.ingimage.com

This book is a translation from the original published under ISBN 978-620-2-24017-8.

Publisher:
Sciencia Scripts
is a trademark of
Dodo Books Indian Ocean Ltd. and OmniScriptum S.R.L publishing group

120 High Road, East Finchley, London, N2 9ED, United Kingdom
Str. Armeneasca 28/1, office 1, Chisinau MD-2012, Republic of Moldova, Europe
Printed at: see last page
ISBN: 978-620-6-10169-7

Contents

Dedications

To my children

Acknowledgements

To Silvina, for her patience and advice.

To my teachers and to all those who, thanks to the knowledge and criteria they taught me, allow me to "make the allowance" every day.

To my current and former colleagues in the Haemotherapy and Immunohaematology Unit, without whose dedication to the blood donor this work would not have been possible. And especially to my Chief, Dr. Estevez, for allowing me to use the service's database.

To my colleagues in "the Network" for being available when an opinion or help is needed so as not to disrupt routine screening or diminish its quality.

To all those who have contributed to the progress in the development of diagnostic techniques for TTIs, whose scientific publications, by a large number of authors dedicated to the investigation of these diseases, have been a reference in the preparation of this thesis.

To my parents, for the education they have given me and the values they have passed on to me.

Glossary

DATA ACQUISITION: acquisition of data using the computer system's own commands.

PROGRAMMATIC AREAS, form of organisation of the Public Health Subsystem, to develop the strategy of primary health care, thinking of it as the gateway to the health system of the community. *(Programmatic Area Department) It* can also be defined as "area of action of a bedside hospital" (*Raya, SM & col, 2017).*

BSI: Intra-hospital Blood Bank.

BLOOD COLLECTIONS: refers to external voluntary blood donation collections. These are a strategy prioritised by the National Blood Plan and are used by all Provincial Blood Therapy Centres and Blood Therapy Services. It is a service provided to donors as it takes place at an off-site location. This facilitates the concurrence of donors and the access to the donation, avoiding long journeys and respecting the quality procedures according to the administrative and technical regulations in force in order to be carried out in different environments, outside the usual areas of haemotherapy *(Blood and Blood Products Department)*.

DGEyC: Dirección General de Estadisticas y Censos, GCBA (GCABA).

TRANSIENTLY DEFERRED DONOR: A donor who was deferred but after a prudential time for the cause of the deferral to subside can be accepted, e.g. a person in asthma crisis cannot donate, but when the asthma subsides and the person does not show symptoms of asthma, he/she can donate.

FALSE POSITIVE DONOR A donor with RR screening and a negative confirmatory test.

INITIALLY REACTIVE DONOR (IR): donor who was reactive in at least one of the mandatory screening reactions.

NON-REACTIVE DONOR donor who was non-reactive for all screening reactions

REJECTED DONOR OR DEFERRED DONOR: A donor who does not meet any of the established requirements to donate blood. The length of the deferral will depend on the cause of the deferral, and may be temporary or permanent.

PERMANENTLY REJECTED OR DEFERRED DONOR: a donor with a non-reversible medical cause of rejection, e.g. having suffered from hepatitis B.

.REPEATEDLY REACTIVE (RR) DONOR: IR donor who, by algorithm, had the reactive marker repeated in duplicate and at least one of these repeats was again reactive.

TRUE POSITIVE DONOR: A donor with RR screening and a positive confirmatory test.

SPECIFICITY OF THE REAGENT: indicates the ability of our estimator to give as negative cases the cases that are really healthy; proportion of correctly identified healthy cases. E=VN/(VN+FP)

GCABA: Government of the Autonomous City of Buenos Aires *(Buenos Aires, city).*

HGAJAF: Hospital General de Agudos Juan A. Fernandez. *(Establishments - Hospitals and Health Centres)*

INDEC: Instituto Nacional de Estad^sticas y Censos (National Institute of Statistics and Census) (*INDEC, Repubiica Argentina)*

ITT: Transfusion-transmitted infections.

PREVALENCE is the number of people suffering from a given event or disease divided by the total population at a given time and place by 10^n .

CUT-OFF POINTS: Value that establishes the Hmite between reactive and non-reactive.

CROSS-REACTION: is the reaction between an antigen and an antibody that was generated against a different but similar antigen.

TRANSFUSIONAL MEDICINE NETWORK, which depends on the General Direction of Hospitals, is integrated by 25 Haemotherapy Services of the Hospitals dependent on the GCABA and a Coordination. Its objective is the conservation and management of human blood resources. For more information: *(Voluntary Blood Donation)*

ENTRIES IN THE DONOR LEDGER: this is each of the entries or lines in the donor ledger. This entry has a unique and unrepeatable number, starting at 1 every first day of the year. They are always correlative and the computerised and paper books coincide. Each entry can correspond to a donor received (whether he/she has donated or not) or to a unit coming from the Network.

SENSITIVITY OF THE REAGENT: indicates the ability of the reagent to give as positive cases the cases that are really diseased; proportion of correctly identified diseased cases. S= PV/(VP+FN)

SEROREACTIVITY percentage of repeatedly reactive (RR) cases over studied.

ECLIPSE WINDOW: The eclipse window is defined as the time between the entry of the **micro-organism** into the body and the time when it is detectable in circulation by highly sensitive direct methods such as molecular biology.

SEROLOGICAL WINDOW: the period until circulating antibodies against that micro-organism start to be detected.

GREY ZONE: Values of an immunoassay reading below the cut-off point where true negative cannot be discriminated from true positive. It is defined from an ROC curve.

Technical summary

This is a descriptive, observational, cross-sectional and retrospective study carried out at the Transfusion Transmissible Infections Laboratory (ITT) of the Haemotherapy and Immunohematology Unit of the General Hospital of Acute Diseases Juan. A. Fernandez belonging to the GCABA. The purpose of this work is to study the average prevalence of compulsory screening diseases in blood and platelet donors, in accordance with the requirements of the National Blood Law and its regulations. This study, which was carried out on 44244 first-time donations made during the period 2006-2017, allows us to characterise this population according to the variables sex, age, place of residence and origin according to birth of the donors.

This provides new health knowledge for the prevention and detection of TTI cases, leading to preventive interventions for new cases and access to specific treatment and follow-up for those affected. It is also useful for the planning of resources needed for such interventions.

Introduction

There are many infectious diseases that have in common an asymptomatic stage in their evolution in which the person can be the transmitting agent of the infection. If, in addition, one of the possible routes of transmission for this infection is blood, its components or derivatives, public health problems are generated. This is shown by numerous pioneering works such as those of Schmunis *(1999)*, Truelove *(1947)*, Moore *(1953)* and Wood *(1955)*.

Transfusion is a perfect route for the spread of diseases that can be transmitted by contact with infected blood, which is why the World Health Organisation *(WHO/WHO, 1999; WHO/WHO, 2005; PAHO/CHA/HT/13.01/WHO, 2013; WHO/HSE/PED/HIP/GHP, 2012; WHO, 2017; Cruz, JR, 2012)* recommends TTI screening in blood banks as a methodology to cut the chain of transmission of TTIs. Therefore, each country has determined based on different parameters (prevalence and incidence, *(Real Delor & col, 2016; Amegeiras & col, 2013; Vladimirsky & col, 2013; Nascimento & col, 2008; Zambrano Plata & Cortez, 2001; Monge-Maillo & col, 2009; Patino Bedoya & col, 2012; Serrano Machuca & col, 2009; Alonso S & col, 2019; Sanodze & col s, 2015; Fay & col, 2005; Angeleri P* & col, sf; Gonzalez & col, 2013; Paz & col, 2013; PAHO, 2017; Stienlauf & col, 2009; Karimi & col, 2017; Posada-Vergara & col, 2006; Biglione & Berin, 2013; Irfan & col, 2013; Abbas Zaheer & col, *2014; Gendler & col, 2011; Riveron Corteguera, 2002; Arrizabalaga, 2000; Department of Health Systems and Services, 2016; (Suarez Larreinaga & Berdasquera Corcho, 2000; Hofstraat & col, 2017; Rabinovich & col, 2017; Kim & col, 2006; Barin, 2000), technical* possibilities *(Biglione & Berin, 2013; CDC/PAHO, 2011; Fainboim H & col, 2013; Bouzas & col, 2013; (Wick & col, 1895; Aach & col, 1981; Welch & col s, 2016; Lia & col, 2018; Mori & col, 2017; Busch, 2004; (Kim & col, 2006; (Mazeron, 2000; Faddy & col, 2016; (Reesink & col, 2010; Liumbruno & Franchin, 2015; Musso & col, 2014),* cost/benefit) *(Ramos-Ligonio & col, 2006; Gendler & Estevez, 2017; Mazeron, 2000; Arbeitskreis Blut, Untergruppe "Bewertung Blutassoziierter Krankheitserreger", 2010)* the mandatory screening of different TTIs in blood banks. The legislation of Argentina *(Law 22990/1983, Decree 1338/04, Ministerial Resolution 797/13, RM 139/14, RM 1507/15, Law 23798/90, Law 22360/80)* in general and of CABA *(Law No. 3.328/09, Decree No. 087/010)* in particular, establishes mandatory screening.

There is a large literature documenting different strategies to prevent transfusion transmission of SIfilis, *(Gonzalez & col, 2015; Fakile & col, 2018)*, Brucellosis *(Gendler S. , 2013; Lucero, NE, 1994; Coppola, 2001; Tsegay & col, 2017)*, *Chagas disease* *(Morales, 1996; law 26281/07; Gendler & Trinca, 2015; Ministerio de*

Salud de la Nacion, 2012; Angheben & col, 2015; Rodrigues Coura, 2015; Cura EN & col , 1992; Sguassero & col, 2015), hepatitis B *(Bouzas, MB & col, sf.)* and C *(Cetiner & col, 2017; Tillmann, 2014; Khan & col, 2017; Morgan Freiman & col, 2016; Gendler S. , 2005),* HIV *(Lya TD & col, 2004; PIWOWAR-MANNING & col, 2015 ; Gendler & Pascuccio, 2007; Gendler S. & col, 2014)* and HTLV *(Berini & col, 2008; Thorstensson & col, 2002)* applied to blood donations (or their components).

The hospitals of the GCABA receive blood donations from people who go to the BSI that exist in them or who go to collections (in public places or private or public institutions) organised by the Red de Medicina Transfusional dependent on the Ministry of Health of CABA. All of them, despite being asymptomatic and apparently healthy *(Sanchez Frenes & col, 2012)* may suffer from infectious diseases and be unaware of their condition.

The mandatory serological and/or molecular screening markers, whose technical characteristics have changed according to technological advances *(Resolution 797/13, RM 139/14, RM 1507/15),* are tested on blood samples *taken* in pilot tubes at the time of donation (see Annex 1: Blood bank workflow). If at least one of these markers is reactive, the unit is discarded and the donor is summoned to report the finding.

It is worth clarifying that before accepting the potential donor for the act of donation, he/she is subjected to a clinical medical questionnaire (see Annex 2: Clinical medical interview form of the Blood Banks of the GCABA Hospitals.), standardised by the National Blood Plan in 2006 through ministerial resolutions, updated in 2013 and 2015 *(RM 1509/2015),* and taken by the Red de Medicina Transfusional del GCABA to create a unified form that is used in all the BSI of ësta jurisdiction to detect the risk of having contracted any TTI (*RM 1507/15),* . This form collects (annex 2), among other donor data, the donor's place of birth (in the presumption that due to population migration or travel we may be dealing with people who were at some stage of their lives in endemic areas for any of the mandatory screening diseases) and current address in order to be able to summon them and inform them of any anomaHa detected in the TTI screening. It also contains a series of questions that ask about different activities that increase the risk of contracting TTIs. If the result of this questionnaire (which includes a blood pressure, temperature and haemoglobin check) is negative, the candidate is accepted as a donor and after the donation will be subjected to the mandatory screening described above (see Annex 3: General workflow of the Donors sector of the blood bank).

WHO/PAHO recommends that in order to reduce the discarding of donated blood, work should be done on two fronts simultaneously *(Schmunis & Cruz, 2005, WHO/PAHO, 2014)*: the quality of the donor, who should be encouraged to be an altruistic and repeat volunteer, and the quality of TTI screening, which depends, among other factors, on the sensitivity and specificity of the chosen method.

The detection of a True Positive donor for each of the 7 diseases being studied represents a possibility of preventing transmission, preventing the appearance of new cases in transfusion recipients and allowing the infected donor (from one patient to another) to be treated and his or her disease, depending on which one it is, to be cured or at least not to progress and not to spread among his or her relatives or sexual contacts. It is therefore important to know how the prevalence of each of these infectious diseases has evolved in our environment.

CHAPTER 1

Objectives

a) General:

To know the total prevalence of the diseases of obligatory screening according to the Blood Law and its regulations, in the Blood and/or Platelet Donors studied in the intrahospital blood bank (BSI) of the Htal Fernandez (from now on they will be called "donors").

b) Spetfficos

- To measure the annual prevalence of each of the above diseases over the period 2006-2017 in donors.
- To characterise these donors according to the following variables: age, sex, declared address, place of birth.
- Describe the co-infections present in these donors.

Design:

Observational, descriptive, cross-sectional, retrospective,

Population and sample:

a) Universe:

Blood and/or platelet donors who came to donate to the BSI of all GCABA Hospitals or to all collections of the Transfusion Medicine Network of the GCABA in the period 2006-2017.

b) Population:

Blood and/or platelet donors who came, in the period 2006-2017, to donate to the BSI of the HGAJAF of the GCABA or to collections organised by ëste hospital and/or by the Red de Medicina Transfusional del GCABA and the units obtained in these collections together with their medical-clinical interview forms were sent to the HGAJAF for study and processing[1] .

c) Units of analysis:

Blood and/or platelet donors at the BSI of the HGJAF or in collections organised by the BSI or the Red de Medicina Transfusional del GCABA in the period 2006-2017 and were repeatedly reactive in the ITT screening.

---

[1] It is clarified that the units were destined to the BSI of HGAJAF because the "Network" determines to which BSI, of the public hospitals of the GCABA, will send the units of blood that are extracted in the collections that it organises. It may be that some, all or none of them reach the HGJAF.

d) Sample:

No sample was taken. The total population of donors studied in the period 2006-2017 was analysed.

e) Inclusion criteria:

1. Requirements to be accepted as a donor of blood or blood components for which it is necessary:

1.1. Be between 18 and 65 years of age. If they are under 18, they must have parental consent and if they are over 65, the haemotherapist must assess whether they are in a fit state to carry out the donation.

1.2. You must have passed the questionnaire and the medical/clinical interview,

1.3. Have completed the donation process.

2. Meet the case definition to be considered True Positive for the period studied and the disease in question.

f) Exclusion criteria

- Donors who do not meet the criteria set out in Ministerial Resolutions 797/13, 139/14. 1507/15.
- Repeatedly Reactive (RR) donors for any of the markers studied that do not meet the definition of true positive for each disease.

g) Elimination criteria:

- Units provided by the Transfusion Medicine Network from other BSI, therefore not screened at HGJAF.
- Donors with incomplete, illegible or erroneous filiation data in the Donor Book of the service's computerised management system.
- Units corresponding to therapeutic bleeding of patients with polyglobulia.
- Donations that met the inclusion and exclusion criteria but did not correspond to a first presentation to donate in this BSI.

CHAPTER 2

Materials and methods

a) Variables:

In the donors accepted for the study, the variables donor without/with ITT x, place of birth, domicile, age and sex were analysed. The definitions of these variables and their characteristics can be found in table 1.

Variable name	Role in the study	Theoretical definition	Operational definition	Scale of measurement
Donor with/without ITT x	Depen- dient	Blood donor with positive results for at least one of the 7 TTIs for mandatory screening in blood bank	Possible outcomes: - Positive - Non-positive	nominal
Place of birth		Place of birth of the donor declared at the time of filling in the clinical interview form	Possible categories: CABA, NEA, NOA, central region, Cuyo, Patagonia[2][3], bordering countries, non-bordering America, the rest.	nominal
Address	Independent:	Address declared by the donor at the time of filling in the clinical interview form	Party for Bs. As. province. commune for CABA3	nominal
Age		Donor's age calculated from the date of birth declared at the time of filling in the clinical interview form.	Age =date of birth-date of donation	Discrete numdrica
Sex		sex declared by the donor at the time of filling in the clinical interview form	Male/female	nominal dichotomous

Table 1: Description of the variables to be studied and their definitions

b) Confounding variables

Strategies were defined to reduce, in prevalence calculations, the confounding effect introduced by clerical errors in data entry and the false positive and false negative results of screening reagents. These are shown in table 2.

Type of data analysed	Possible confounder	Element to diminish the effect
ITT screening result	Cross-reactions (reagent	Confirmatory - complementary

[2] The division into regions in Argentina is in line with that of the DEIS in its bulletins *(Dir. de Estad^stica e Information de Salud, Min. de Salud y Desarrollo Social, sf.*

[3] To assign the addresses to the CABA communes, the GCBA commune search engine was used *(Buenos Aires Ciudad, Jefatura de Gabinete, sf).*

	specificity)	reactions Case definition (true positive and false positive)
	Reagent sensitivity / serological window / eclipse window / cut-off point selection	Technological changes/NAT/
	Transcription of data and results into management system	Double check

Table 2: Confounders and strategies to reduce the effect of confounders

c) Equipment, techniques and instruments.

i. Initial databases: There are 2 databases:

(1) **Rhesus (Sistema de Gestion information de Banco de Sangre):** is the computer platform where all the events of the Unidad de Hemoterapia e Inmunohematolog^a del Htal. Gral. de Agudos J, A. Fernandez are uploaded. These events include everything related to blood donation, transfusions, follow-up of pregnant women, etc. For this work we acquired the data, in electronic form, from the Book of Donors corresponding to the period 2006-2017.

(2) **RR Excel file**: this contains the information of all the laboratory tests (screening, confirmatory, complementary) that were performed on each donor who tested RR in at least one screening test. An outline of this file can be seen in Figure 1.

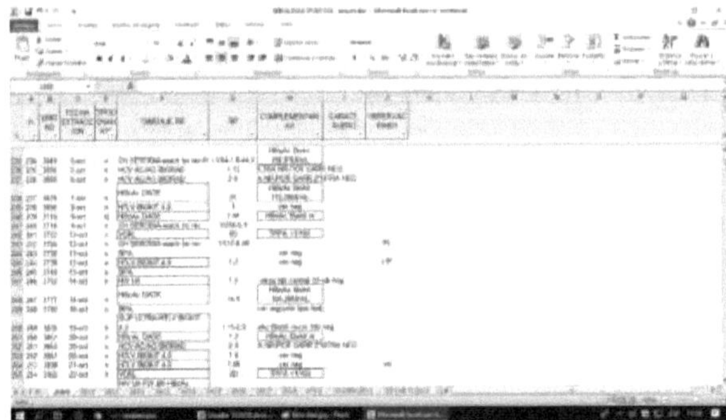

Illustration 1: Partial screenshot of the Excel RR file

ii. Description of the processing of the databases of the site previous:

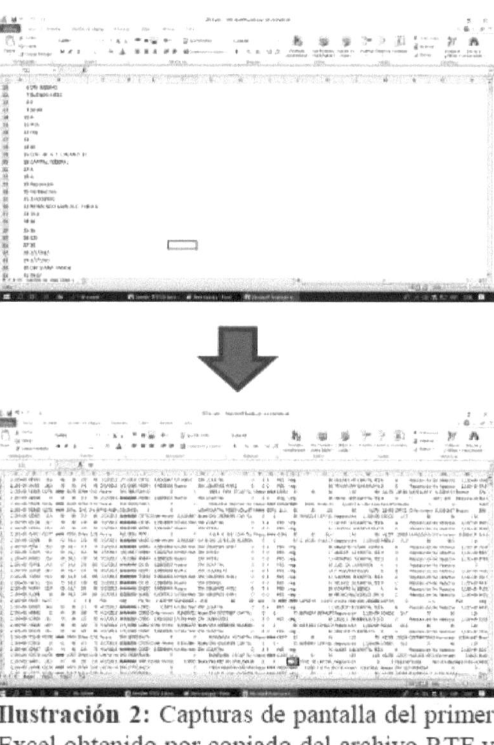

Ilustración 2: Capturas de pantalla del primer Excel obtenido por copiado del archivo RTF y del mismo post encolumnado.

Illustration 2: Screenshots of the first Excel file obtained by copying the RTF file and the same post collated.

(1) **Electronic Donors' Book**: The **Donors' Book** was purchased in RTF text format. This was copied into MS Excel. The database thus obtained had to be subjected to a sorting phase in order to properly collate the different variables (see illustration 2).

(2) **RR Excel file**: Results were copied confirmatory/complementary in the appropriate rows of the database obtained from the Donor Book

(3) **Excel total:** we call the Excel file obtained from the merge as^. of the ordered donor book (ii-1) and the Excel RR (ii-2).

(4) **Database:** the total Excel was cleared of those columns containing data that were not included in the **database:**

- They allow the donor to be identified, in order to meet the ethical requirements of safeguarding the privacy of the persons studied.

- They were not going to be the subject of analysis in this work, as a blood group or a person for whom they donated.

This resulted in a refined database and anonymized, which we call the "**Database**", (Graph

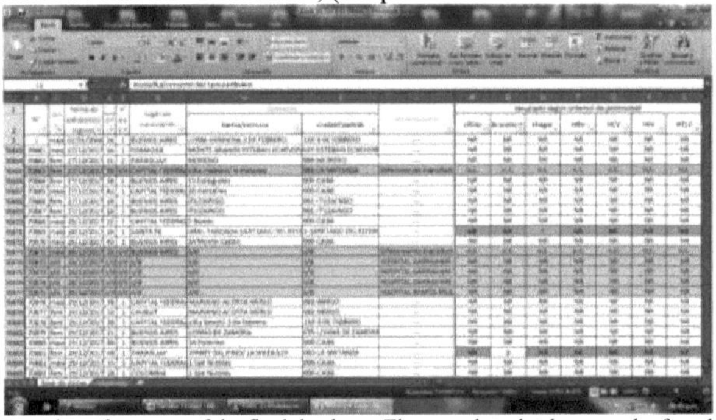

Illustration 3: Screenshot of a sector of the final database. The complete database can be found in annex 1.

(5) **Data analysis**: was performed on the final database, using filters and different MS Excel functions. The results were expressed with summary measures mentioned in table 6 or were, for the most part, plotted with MS Excel. Those that required the use of other software are:

- *Donor's address:* map modification made with Paint
- *Age and sex:* plotted as population pyramids using Epidat 4.2.
- *Diagrams and flowcharts*: made with y-ed

Clarification: The date of donation will be used as a reference for the type of screening method available at that time and for the calculation of age from the date of birth.

111.Laboratory methods used in the period 2006-2017:

a. Screening

Laboratory screening techniques varied over time. Table 3 summarises all methodologies used between 2006 and 2017.

Disease	Scoreboard	Type Reagents used	Reagent method
Sffilis	Rheagmic acids	VDRL usr	flocculation
		VDRL RPR	Binding favoured by carbon particles
Brucellosis	Anti Brucella Ac	BPA	Direct binding
Chagas	Anti T cruzi antibodies	HAI	Indirect agglutination

				of sensitised red blood cells
			APG	Indirect binding of sensitised gelatine particles
			Trypanosome lysate ELISA	Colourimëtric immunoassay
			Recombinant ELISA	Recombinant antigen colourimmunoassay
			chemiluminescence	Luminescent read-through immunoassay of recombinant antigen
HBV hepatitis	Viral antigens	HBsAg	ELISA	Colourimëtric immunoassay
			chemiluminescence	Luminescent read-out immunoassay
		Viral DNA	NAT	Qualitative molecular biology
	Viral antibodies	HBcAc	ELISA	Colourimëtric immunoassay
			chemiluminescence	Luminescent read-out immunoassay
HCV hepatitis	Viral antigens	Core Ag	ELISA	Colorimetric immunoassay
			chemiluminescence	Luminescent read-out immunoassay
		Viral RNA	NAT	Qualitative molecular biology
	Viral antibodies	Ac anti HCV	ELISA	Colorimetric immunoassay
			chemiluminescence	Luminescent read-out immunoassay
	Simultaneous viral antigens and antibodies	Core Ag+ anti-HCV Ac	ELISA4° ELISA4° ELISA4° ELISA4° ELISA4° ELISA4° ELISA4 generation	Colorimetric immunoassay
			Chemiluminiscence4° Chemicals4° Chemicals4° Chemicals4° Chemicals4° Chemicals4° Chemicals4°	Luminescent read-out immunoassay

			Chemicals generation	
HIV/AIDS	Viral antigens	Core Ag	ELISA	Colorimetric immunoassay
			chemiluminescence	Luminescent read-out immunoassay
		Viral RNA	NAT	Qualitative molecular biology
	Viral antibodies	Ac anti HIV	ELISA	Colorimetric immunoassay
			chemiluminescence	Luminescent read-out immunoassay
	Simultaneous viral antigens and antibodies	Core Ag+ anti-HIV Ac	ELISA4° ELISA4° ELISA4° ELISA4° ELISA4° ELISA4° ELISA4 generation	Colorimetric immunoassay
			Chemiluminisce nce4° Chemicals4° Chemicals4° Chemicals4° Chemicals4° Chemicals4° Chemicals4° Chemicals generation	Luminescent read-out immunoassay
ATLL/TSP	Viral antibodies		ELISA	Colorimetric immunoassay
			chemiluminescence	Luminescent read-out immunoassay

Table 3: Reagents used in ITT screening, by disease in different periods. The technical rationale for each reaction is given.

b. Additional evidence:

The complementary/confirmatory reactions done in-house can be seen in table 4 while those that were referred to other centres are shown in table 5.

Disease	Technique used	Basis	Effect
Syphilis	TPPA	Detection of trepondemic Acs	confirmatory
Chagas	ELISA	different from the one used .-4 in the routine	Increase in Positive predictive value
	APG	Detection of Ac	
HBV	HBsAc	ELISA	complementary
HCV	2° Ac ELISA	each brand has a	Increase in

		different recombinant peptide design	Positive predictive value
HIV	Western blot	Detection of Ac on the basis of separated Ag by electrophoresis	confirmatory

Table 4: Description of complementary/confirmatory techniques performed in the ITT laboratory of HGAJAF

Disease	**Referred to**
Brucellosis	ANLIS Malbran, reference centre for brucellosis
HIV	HGAJAF Central Laboratory[4] [5]
HTLV	INBRIS

Table 5 Enumeration of locations to which samples were derived for confirmation.

[4] If the routine Elisa that doubled with the HAI was recombinant, a trypanosome lysate ELISA was performed as the 3rd reaction and vice versa.

[5] When there is a lack of reagents in the ITT laboratory of the HGAF.

CHAPTER 3

Data processing and analysis

a) Definition of a confirmed case:

Based on existing diagnostic algorithms and laboratory tests, the cases considered positive for each of the 7 infections studied were defined as follows:

- **S^filis:** Repeatedly Reactive Reagmic Test (RR) and Reactive TPPA *(Kamb, M & col, 2015)*
- **Brucellosis** Any positive test *(Moral, M & col, 2013)* from the following tests performed by the National Reference Centre (NRC) for Brucellosis (*Lucero, NE & col, 2008)*: complement fixation, tube test (Wright), SAT, CELISA, IELISA
- **Chagas** RR in at least two serological screening techniques irrespective of the titre or the positivity ratio (pr) of the screening result (*Nation's Ministry of Health, 2012)*.
- **HBV** any of the following marker combinations *(Angeleri P, & col, 2016; Fainboim H& col , 2013)*:

o HBsAg RR and/or NAT RR and HBcAc RR

o NAT NR, HBcAc RR and HBsAc RR

o HBsAg NR, HBcAc RR and HBsAc RR

o HBsAg RR, positive neutralisation and all other markers NR

o HBsAg RR and HBsAc RR

- **HCV** any of the following combinations of markers *(Alter M & col, 2003; Angeleri P & col, 2016; Gregoire & col, 2018)*:

o a single anti-HCV RR result of PR greater than the CDC cutoff
or 2 anti-HCV results by different mëtodo, irrespective of the PR

o PCR or NAT reactive (irrespective of serological results)

o HCV core Ag with positive neutralisation (irrespective of serological results).

- **HIV**

or RR screening with 3rd or 4th generation reagents independent of RP and one of the following reactive/positive markers *(Recoder, ML & col, 2016), (PAHO/WHO, 2009), (Gendler & Pascuccio, 2007), (Lya & col, 2004):*

- NAT
- Western Blot
- Neutralisation of Ag P24

o ELISA 3rd generation RP>3 and another antibody technique (APG, rapid test) o p24 RR.

- **HTLV** Western Blot positive NRC for retroviruses *(Berini & col, 2008).*

b) Treatment given to each variable in the database

Variable name	Scale of measurement	Summary measures
Donor without/with ITT x	nominal	Ratios: 1- Total prevalence=N° of those suffering from the event or disease/total population for that period and place x1000 2-Specific rates: equal definition by place of birth, by area of residence, by age range, by sex, by type of donor, by donation period, each expressed with its CI95%.
Date of birth	discrete numërica	It will only be used to calculate age if age was not entered or if there is a calculation error.
Place of birth	nominal	N per category (for Argentinians CABA or region, for foreigners bordering or not bordering country within the continent or outside the continent)
Address	nominal	in CABA (neighbourhoods/communes) and Pcia BA (cities/partido, GBA/non-GBA)
Age	Discrete Numtirica	Mean and median plus interquartile ranges or division into 5-year intervals and histograms.
Sex	nominal dichotomous	N by category, % N by category, % N by category, % N by category, % N by category, % N by category, % N by category, % N by category, % N by category, % N by category, % N by category, %
Donation date	discrete numerics	N/month or N/year

Table 6: Classification of the variables to be studied and their treatment

Resources and schedule of activities

a) Human resources:

Researcher involved in the project: *Bioq.* ***Silvina Alejandra Gendler***

c) Equipment and infrastructure.

1 PC, MS Office package and internet access, 1 pen drive, 1 printer, 3 reams of A4 paper, 4 pens, 1 chair, 1 desk.

d) Ethical and regulatory aspects:

Prior to the field stage, the relevant presentation was made to the HGAJAF's CEI. The investigation was initiated once approval was obtained.

During the processing of the databases, only information that was useful to characterise the donor was taken, avoiding the use of anything that would allow the identification of individual persons, due to the sensitivity of the information handled.

e) Schedule of activities

Description of tasks	MES																				
	4	5	6	7	8	9	10	11	12	1	2	3	4	5	6	7	8	9	10	11	12
Project presentation																					
Literature review																					
Evaluation of instruments																					
Presentation to the HGAJAF's CEI																					
Training of field workers / Fieldworkers	-	-	-	-	-	-	-	-	-	-	-	-	-	-	-	-	-	-	-	-	-
Redaction of progress report																					
Codification.																					
Data processing, data analysis																					
Redaction of final report																					

Table 7: Timeline of activities carried out

CHAPTER 4

Results:

a) Entries in the Electronic Management System Donor Ledger

In the period 2007-2018 a total of 70892 registrations were made in the Donor Book. The inclusion/exclusion/elimination criteria reduced these records to a final population of 44244 donors eligible for this study (see Graphol). The remainder is composed of 7698 units provided by the Transfusion Medicine Network, 15556 donors who were deferred, temporarily or permanently, and 3394 due to incomplete/eligible filiatory data or because they were not the first donation studied in this service (see graphs 2 and 3).

As can be seen in table 8, deferrals increase sharply between 2009 and 2010. This is due to a change in the service's working methods from that year onwards. Until that time, only deferrals due to causes related to the collection of the blood unit (lipotimia, clogged needle, etc.) were recorded in the computer system, and from 2010 all deferrals during the medical-clinical interview were added, so that the figures for the first 3 years would not be comparable to the rest.

It should also be mentioned that the drop, in the same table, of the number in the last year in the column "Eligible donors", was due to a new regulation *(RM 1508/17)* in force from that year onwards, which requires replacement donors to be required from patients, whether they require transfusion support or not.

Records in the donor book

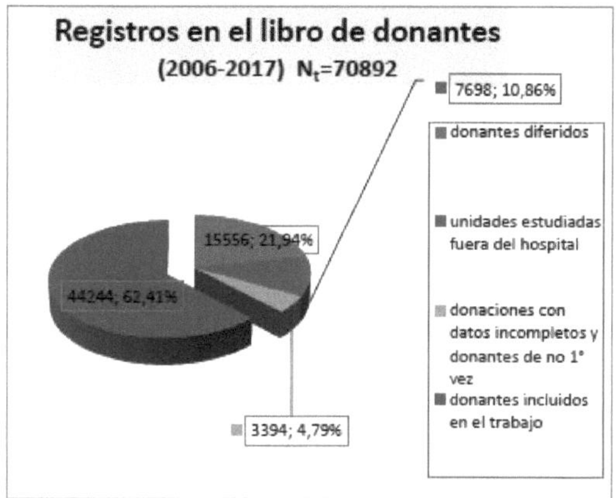

■ 7698; 10,86%
■ deferred donors
■ units studied outside the hospital
■ donations with incomplete data and donors of no 1°.
This time
■ donors included in the work

Graph 1: Total donor book entries between 2006 and 2017 by source of production. For each of the 4 categories the amount (N) and the percentage it represents of the total income is reported.

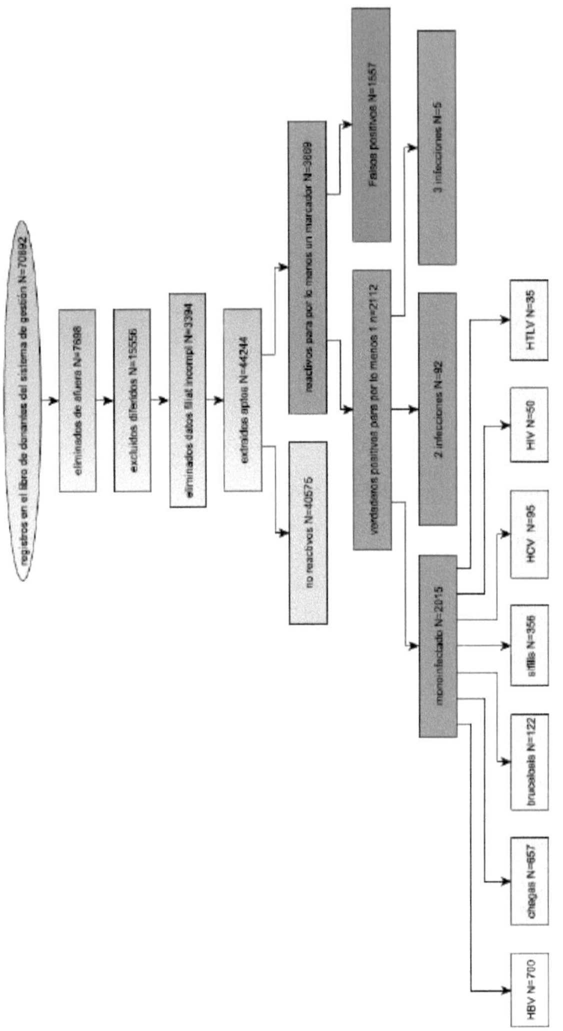

Figure 2: Total entries in the Donor Book according to inclusion/exclusion/elimination criteria and the classification of donors included in the study.

Ano	Eliminated		Excluded	Including	Total
	Units studied in other centres	Discarded extracted donors	Deferred donors	Eligible donors removed	
2006	671	124	150	4000	4945
2007	650	227	127	4297	5301
2008	643	281	130	4446	5500
2009	459	335	129	3917	4840
2010	505	313	1264	3987	6069
2011	940	308	1623	3293	6164
2012	794	319	1646	3260	6019
2013	1037	273	1857	3145	6312
2014	279	365	2054	4543	7241
2015	451	308	3145	3744	7648
2016	568	283	2097	3219	6167
2017	701	258	1334	2393	4686
Sum	***7698***	***3394***	***15556***	***44244***	***70892***
Average	607,38	274,45	758,39	3632,57	5844,12
Std. dev.	212,84	61,81	980,86	636,03	916,25
Max.	1037	124	3145	3917	7648
Min.	451	227	127	2393	5301

Table 8: Total records in the donor book between 2006 and 2017 according to their source of production by year.

b) Characteristics of the study population:

Hereafter, the characteristics of the 44244 donors meeting the inclusion/exclusion/elimination criteria will be discussed.

a. Mandatory TTIs studied

i. Positive cases

Applying the case definition (see section 7-a) for each of the 7 infections of compulsory screening in the Blood Bank, 385 cases of s^filis, 129 cases of Brucellosis, 713 cases of Chagas disease, 776 cases of HBV infection, 111 cases of hepatitis C, 58 cases of HIV positive and 42 cases of HTLV infection were counted. The distribution of cases by year can be seen in table 9. At this point it should be clarified that for the period 2006-2008 there was no possibility of confirming brucellosis and therefore no cases are reported for that period.

INFECCION	AÑO												Total
	2006	2007	2008	2009	2010	2011	2012	2013	2014	2015	2016	2017	
sifilis	32	31	44	11	15	18	33	32	52	52	40	25	385
brucelosis	s/d*	s/d	s/d	9	10	12	7	11	23	23	11	23	129
chagas	85	94	88	58	61	45	46	35	62	66	50	23	713
HBV	79	66	80	74	73	55	80	56	58	55	54	46	776
HCV	17	19	12	7	12	11	7	3	4	6	9	4	111
HIV	6	3	9	4	7	6	3	2	9	6	0	3	58
HTLV	4	3	4	8	2	1	1	3	6	4	3	3	42

Table 9: Number of positives for each of the 7 infections studied per year.

ii. Total prevalence

Starting from the geometrical formula:

persons suffering from a specific disease n
P= л 10 for that time y place
total population

(see glossary and table 6) the total prevalence of each mandatory screening TTI was calculated as the number of true positive cases out of the 44244 total donors studied. The exception to this calculation was Brucellosis. In this case, as it was not possible to discriminate true positives from false positives in the first 3 years, as explained above, donors in those years were excluded from the total prevalence calculation. Therefore the denominator was reduced to 31501 donors for that TTI. See table 9 and graph 3.

iii. Annual prevalence

The annual prevalence results for each of the 7 infections studied, expressed per 1000 donors, and their variation over the study period are presented below (graphs 4 to 10 and table 10).

ITT	Average annual prevalence	Desv. Stand.
Syphilis	8,80	3,43
Brucellosis	4,26	2,39
Chagas	15,70	3,80
HBV	17,73	2,95
HCV	2,46	1,17
HIV	1,27	0,63
HTLV	0,94	0,48

Table 10: Average annual prevalences for each ITT expressed per 1000 donors

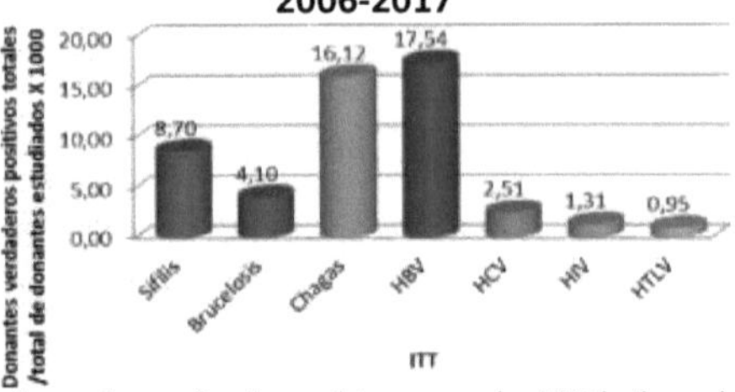

Figure 4: Total prevalence of each mandatory screening TTI in the period 2006-2017

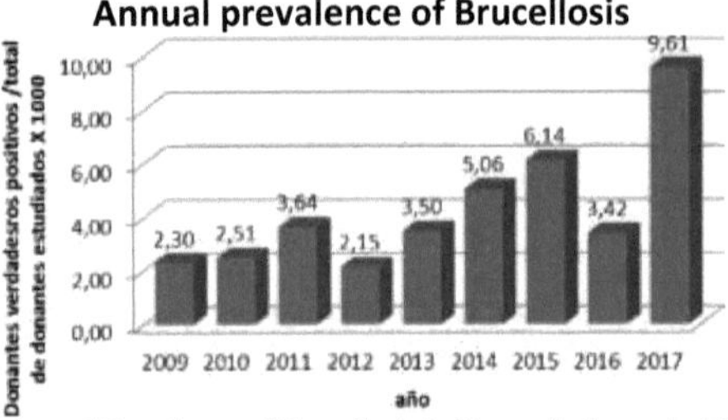

Figure 5: Annual Prevalence of Brucellosis in Donors in the period 2009-2017

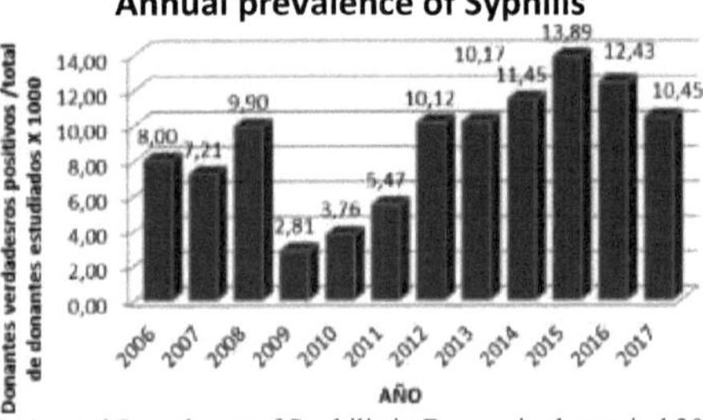

Figure 3: Annual Prevalence of Syphilis in Donors in the period 2006-2017

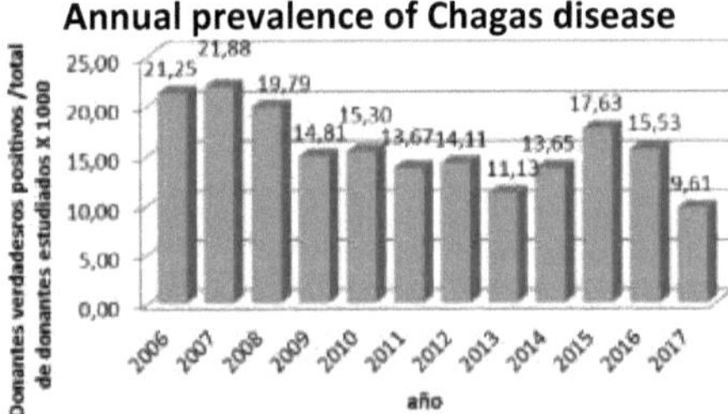

Figure 6: Annual prevalence of Chagas disease in donors in the period 2006-2017

Annual prevalence of HBV infection

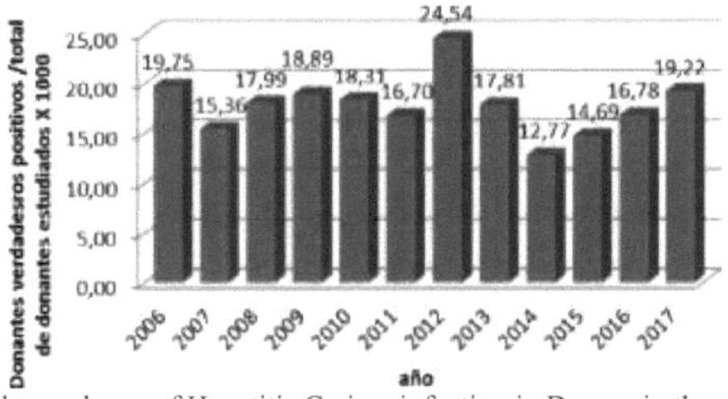

Figure 7: Annual prevalence of Hepatitis C virus infection in Donors in the period 2006-2017

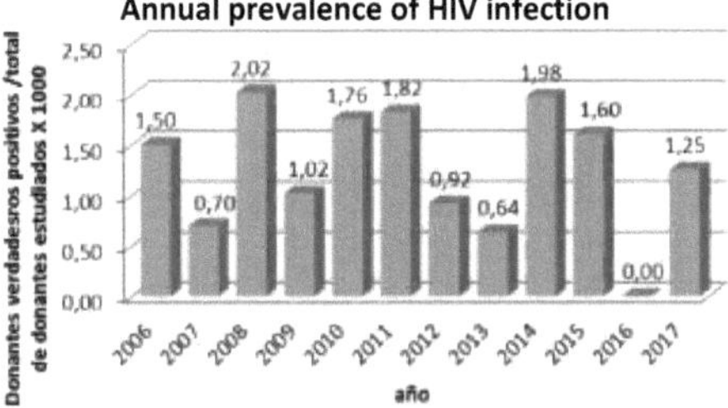

Figure 9: Annual prevalence of Human Immunodeficiency Virus infection in Donors in the period 2006-2017

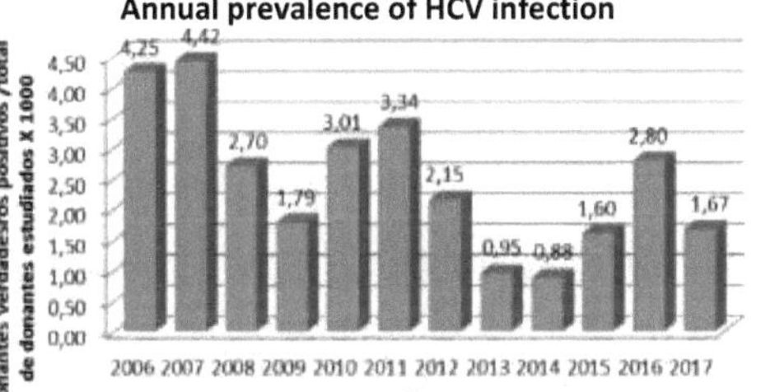

Figure 8: Annual prevalence of Hepatitis C virus infection in Donors in the period 2006-2017

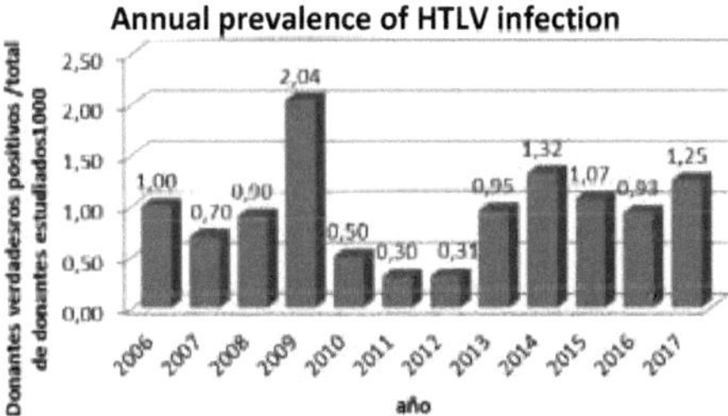

Figure 10: Annual Prevalence of Human T Lymphotropic Virus Infection in Donors 2006-2017

b. Distribution of donors by age and sex:

The age averages (table 10) for each of the groups of positives do not show a noticeable difference between sexes but in several cases the median and/or mode are different, which speaks of an age/sex distribution with its own characteristics for each ITT.

The male/female ratio varies from a minimum of 1.39 for Brucellosis to a maximum of 3.83 for HIV and 2.47 for the total population studied. For Syphilis it is 2.74, for Chagas 3.60 and for HBV, HCV and HTLV it is 3.19, 2.08 and 2.50 respectively.

Table 10 shows the mean, median and mode values for each sex in each ITT.

Figures 11 to 20 show the distribution of donors (total or positive as appropriate) by quintiles according to sex. Figures 11 and 12 were not constructed based on the results of this research, but are added as a reference for further discussion. Since 99.41% of donors are domiciled in CABA or Buenos Aires province, the first graph was made by adding the populations of Buenos Aires province and CABA based on data from the 2010 Population Census *(Inst. Nac. de Estad^sticas y Censos, 2010)*, taking only the quintiles that correspond to people eligible to donate blood, according to the law (i.e. 18 to 65 years old). This graph shows a population with slight ageing trends, where there is no evidence of a predominance of one sex over the other.

The next graph, which is consistent with a young population, corresponds to deferred donors, i.e. those who were not in a position to donate. Here again, there is no gender predominance.

Figure 13, which represents the donors who were enrolled in this study. This graph shows that the male population becomes predominant, maintaining the pattern of a young population. The predominance of the male sex over the female sex is maintained for the positives of the different TTIs studied, although in each case different age distributions are presented.

Sex		M	F
Total donors	half	35,9	36,4
	median	34	35
	mode	28	26
	N	31498	12746
Syphilis	half	39,0	37,1
	median	37	36
	mode	37	23
	N	282	103
Brucellosis	half	35,5	32,3
	median	36	30,5
	mode	26	24
	N	75	54
Chagas	half	42,3	42,3
	median	41	44
	mode	38	36
	N	558	155
HBV	half	40,0	39,4
	median	39	39
	mode	38	24
	N	591	185
HCV	half	43,5	37,0
	median	43	38
	mode	35	27
	N	75	36
HIV	half	35,7	38,2
	median	35,5	37,5
	mode	34	47
	N	46	12
HTLV	half	36,8	41,2
	median	36	39
	mode	32	60
	N	30	12

Table 11: Total cases, mean, median and mode of ages for all screened donors and for ITT-positive donors separated by sex.

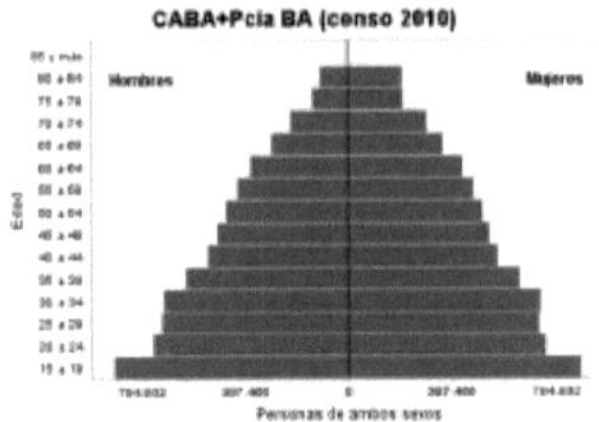

Gráfico 11:-Sumatoria de la población de CABA y provincia de Buenos Aires según censo 2010 por quintiles y sexo.

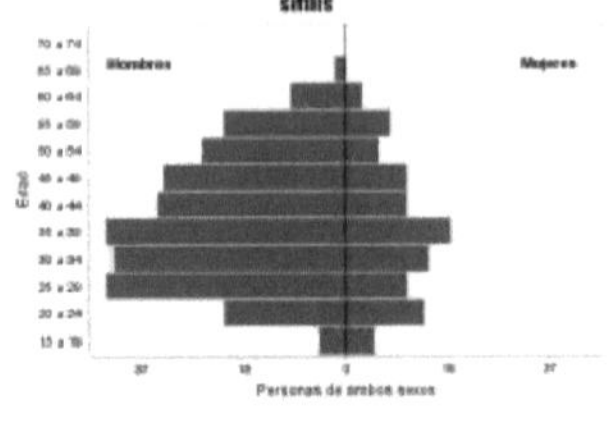

Gráfico 14: Donantes positivos para Sífilis por quintiles y sexo para el periodo 2006-2017.

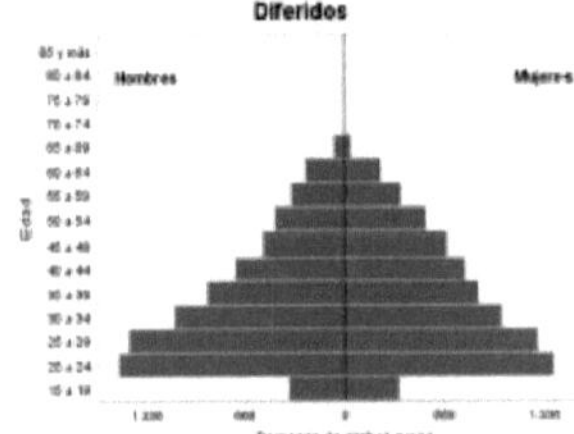

Gráfico 12: Donantes diferidos realizadas en el BSI del HGAJAF y en donaciones recibidas de colectas de la Red de Medicina Transfusional del GCABA por quintiles de edad y sexo para el periodo 2006-2017.

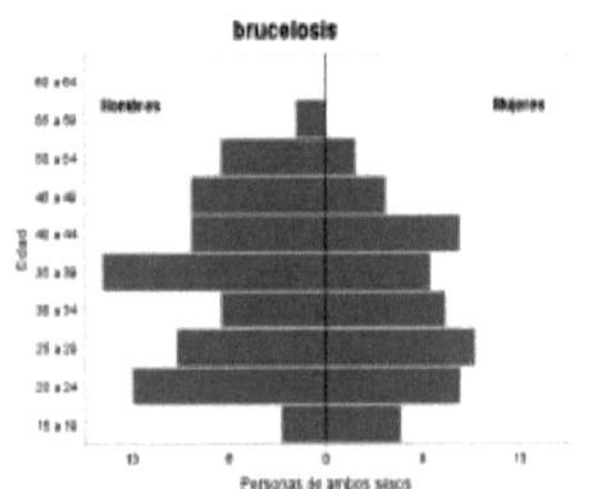

Gráfico 15: Donantes positivos para Brucelosis por quintiles de edad y sexo para el periodo 2006-2017.

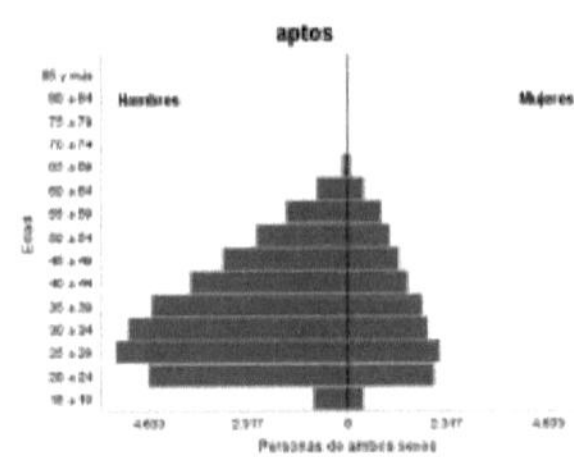

Gráfico 13:-Donantes aptos según los criterios de inclusión/exclusión/eliminación por quintiles de edad y sexo para el periodo 2006-2017.

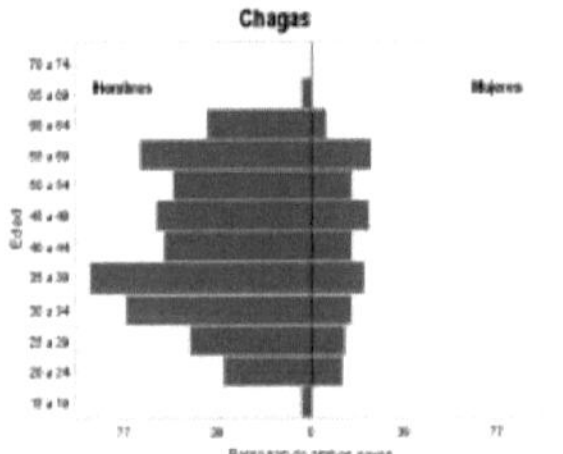

Gráfico 16: Donantes positivos para Chagas por quintiles de edad y sexo para el periodo 2006-2017.

Figure 11:- Population of CABA and province of Buenos Aires according to the 2010 census by quintiles and sex.
Figure 12: Deferred donors made at the BSI of HGAJAF and donations received from collections of the Red de Medicina Transfusional del GCABA by age quintiles and sex for the period 2006-2017.
Figure 13: Eligible donors according to inclusion/exclusion/elimination criteria by age quintiles and sex for the period 2006-2017.
Figure 14: Sphilis-positive donors by quintile and sex for the period 2006-2017.
Figure 15: Brucellosis positive donors by age quintiles and sex for the period 2006-2017.

Figure 16: Chagas-positive donors by age quintiles and sex for the period 2006-2017.

Figure 17: HBV-positive donors by age quintiles and sex for the period 2006-2017.
Figure 19: HIV-positive donors by age quintile and sex for the period 2006-2017.

Figure 18: HCV positive donors by age quintiles and sex for the period 2006-2017.
Figure 20: HTLV-positive donors by age quintiles and sex for the period 2006-2017.

c. Distribution of donors by place of birth

The donors studied at the BSI of the J. A. Fernandez Hospital in the period 2006-2017 were classified according to their place of birth. For this purpose, the division into regions of our country proposed by the DEIS was used (see Map 1). CABA was put as a separate category. Foreigners were grouped into those belonging to neighbouring countries,

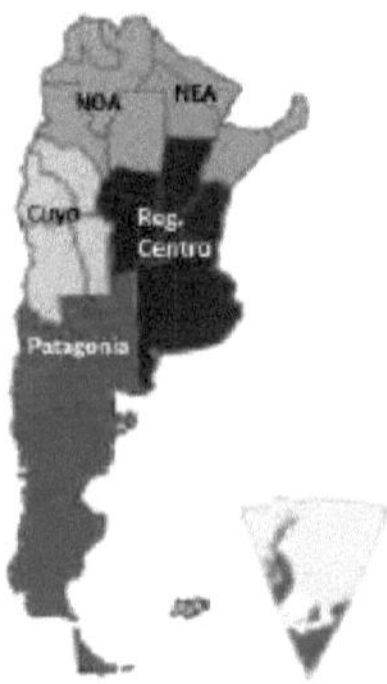

Map 1: Geographical regions into which the Argentine provinces are grouped according to the DEIS bulletins *(Ministry of Health, Argentina, n.d.).*

Americans from non-border countries and the rest of the world. The results are shown in graph 21

Using the same criteria, positive donors for each ITT for the same period and location were plotted (graphs 22 to 28). Table 12 shows the total data by place of birth and positive marker.

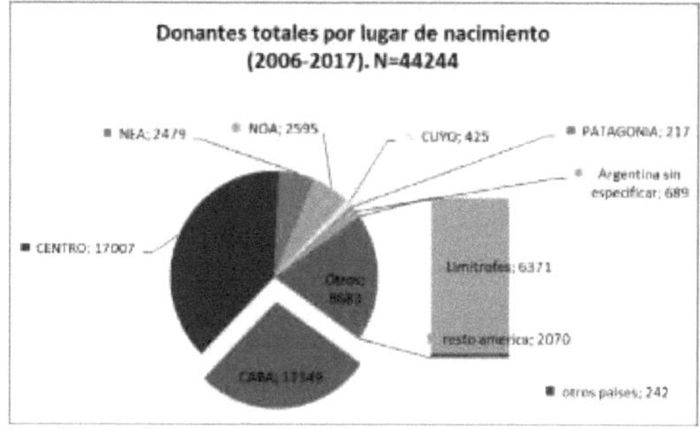

Figure 21: Distribution of donors by place of birth. The name of the region is indicated y the total number of studied.

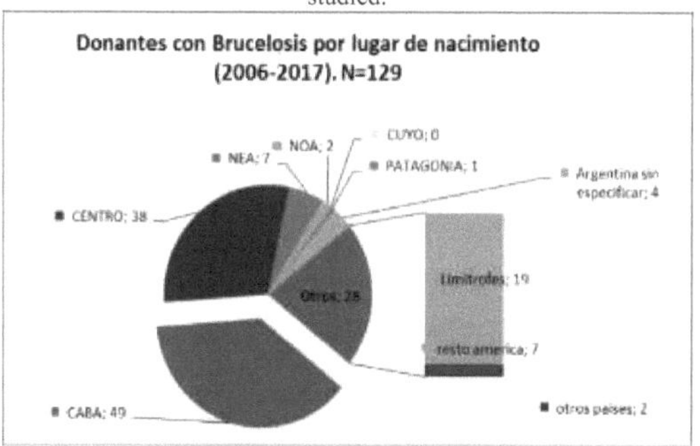

Figure 23: Distribution of Brucellosis positive donors by place of birth. The name of the region is indicated y the total number of tested.

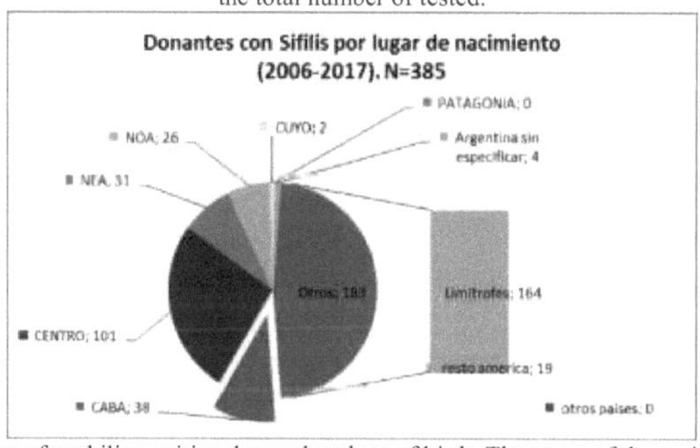

Figure 22: Distribution of syphilis-positive donors by place of birth. The name of the region is indicated and the total number studied.

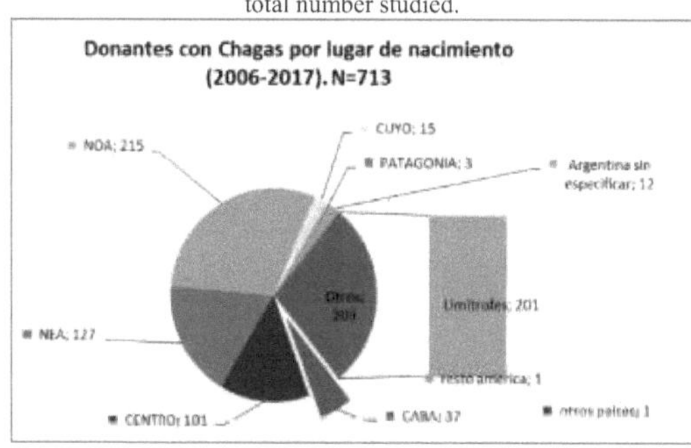

Figure 24: Distribution of Chagas-positive donors by place of birth. The name of the region and the total number of people studied are indicated.

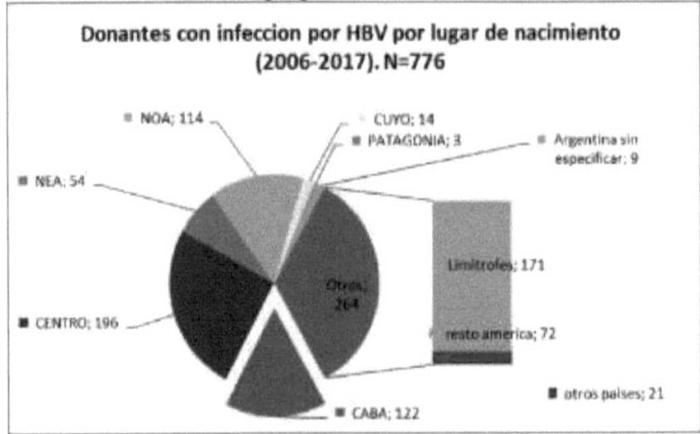

Figure 25: Distribution of HBV-positive donors by place of birth. The name of the region is indicated y the total number of tested donors.

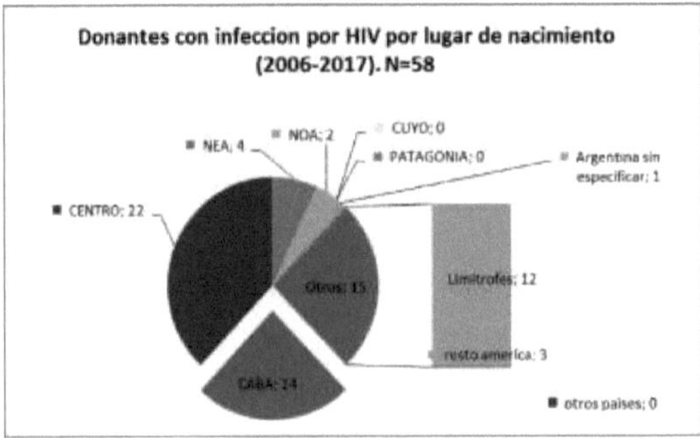

Figure 27: Distribution of HIV-positive donors by place of birth. The name of the region is indicated y the total number of tested.

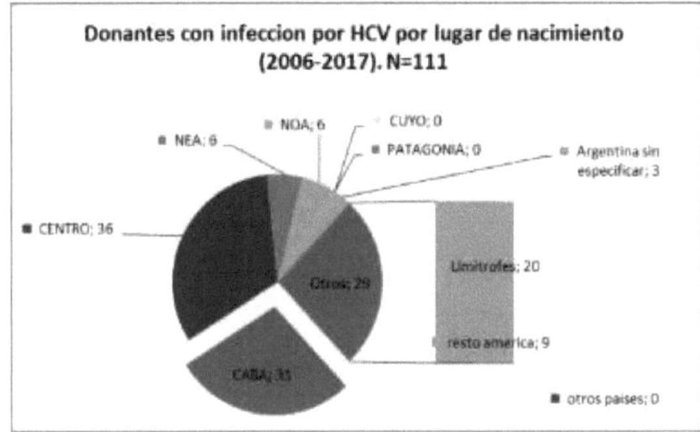

Figure 26: Distribution of HCV-positive donors by place of birth. The name of the region and the total number studied are indicated.

Donors with HTLV infection by place of birth (2006-2017).
place of birth (2006-2017). N=42

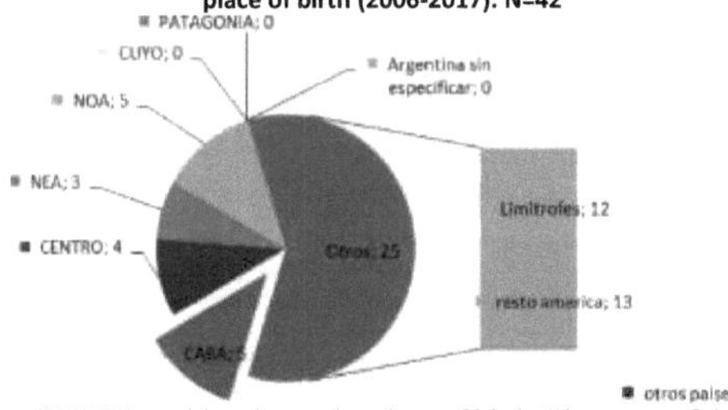

Figure 28: Distribution of HTLV-positive donors by place of birth. The name of the region is indicated y the total number of studied donors.

Region	Provincia	Total donan-tes	Sifilis	Bruce-losis	Chagas	HBV	HCV	HIV	HTLV
CABA		12149	38	49	37	122	31	14	5
CENTRO	BUENOS AIRES	15632	88	32	75	166	31	19	4
	CORDOBA	358	3	3	6	11	3	1	
	SANTA FE	384	6	2	13	11	1	1	
	ENTRE RIOS	581	4	1	6	8	1	1	
	LA PAMPA	52			1				
NEA	CORRIENTES	734	7	2	22	8	1	3	
	MISIONES	698	10		8	22	1		2
	CHACO	692	8	3	77	14	4	1	1
	FORMOSA	355	6	2	20	9			
NOA	JUJUY	474	2	1	15	45		1	3
	SALTA	507	5		27	43	1		2
	TUCUMAN	669	10	1	28	10	2		
	SANTIAGO DEL ESTERO	763	6		135	6	1		
	CATAMARCA	131	1		9	7	1		
	LA RIOJA	51	2		1	3	1	1	
CUYO	MENDOZA	229			7	6			
	SAN JUAN	124	2		5	6			
	SAN LUIS	72			3	2			
PATAGO-NIA	RIO NEGRO	52			2	1			
	NEUQUEN	54				1			
	SANTA CRUZ	37		1	1	1			
	CHUBUT	62							
	TIERRA DEL FUEGO	12				1			
Argentina sin especificar		689	4	4	12	9	3	1	
Limítrofes	URUGUAY	496	6	1	2	20	3	1	
	BRASIL	118			1	3			
	PARAGUAY	4610	149	15	94	103	14	10	9
	BOLIVIA	965	9	2	104	42	1	1	2
	CHILE	182		1		3	2		1
RESTO SUDAMERICA	PERU	1734	17	5	1	67	8	3	13
	COLOMBIA	259	1	1		3	1		
	ECUADOR	3							
	VENEZUELA	3							
RESTO AMERICA	CUBA	38	1	1		1			
	Rep. DOMINICANA	3				1			
	NICARAGUA	1							
	MEXICO	1							
	USA	27							
	CANADA	1							
EUROPA	ALEMANIA	40				3			
	AMSTERDAM	15				2			
	ESPAÑA	55		1	1	1			
	FRANCIA	13							
	GRECIA	2				1			
	ITALIA	47				1			
	SUIZA	1							
	RUMANIA	1							
	RUSIA	9				1			
	UCRANIA	17		1		2			
CERCANO ORIENTE	ARMENIA	1				1			
	TURQUIA	8							
	IRAN	1							
	ISRAEL	1							
	EGIPTO	1							
	ARGELIA	1							
LEJANO ORIENTE	JAPON	1							
	TAIWAN	5				2			
	CHINA	13				5			
	COREA	8				2			
	FILIPINAS	2							
suma		44244	385	129	713	776	111	58	42

Table 12: Donors by place of birth

d. Distribution of donors by address

In order to geographically locate the Intra-Hospital Blood Bank, where the work was carried out, map 2 shows the political division of CABA, according to the law of communes *(law 1777/05)*, superimposed with the division by **Programmatic Areas**.

In this map the programme area corresponding to Htal Fernandez is coloured. This area includes commune 14 (Palermo), commune 2 (Recoleta) and the Retiro neighbourhood, which is one of the six that make up commune 1. This last neighbourhood includes one of the most important slums in the city in terms of number of inhabitants.

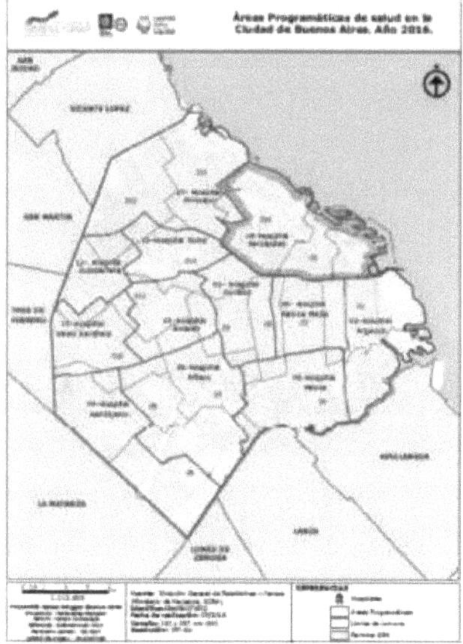

Map 2: Location of the programme area corresponding to Htal Fernandez is coloured in yellow (DGEyC, GCABA, *(Dir. Gral. de Estad^sticay Censos, GCABA, 2016).*

CABA, in turn, is surrounded by an urban agglomerate called Greater Buenos Aires (GBA), which belongs to the province of the same name. The GBA was delimited by provincial law *(Legislature of the Province of Buenos Aires, 2006)* with the aim, among others, of decentralising the administration of the most populous districts. The bibliography shows different ways of grouping the districts that make up the GBA, as shown in maps 3 and 4. In the first, the municipalities closest to CABA are divided into three geographical zones: North, West and South. In the second map, the districts are divided into 4 concentric crowns or cordons.

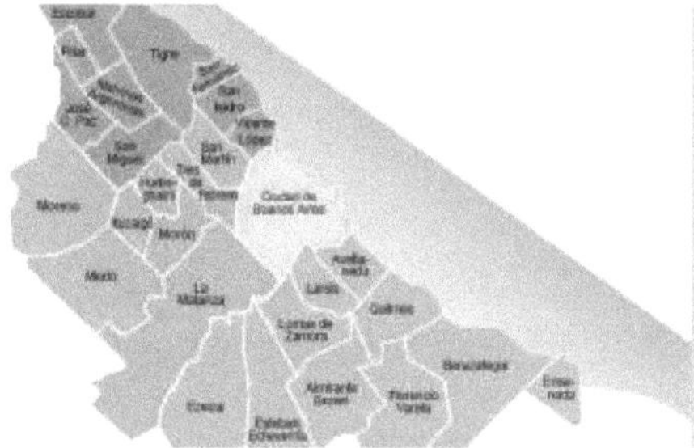

Map 3: Partidos of Greater Buenos Aires showing the north, west and south (*El cronista, sf)*

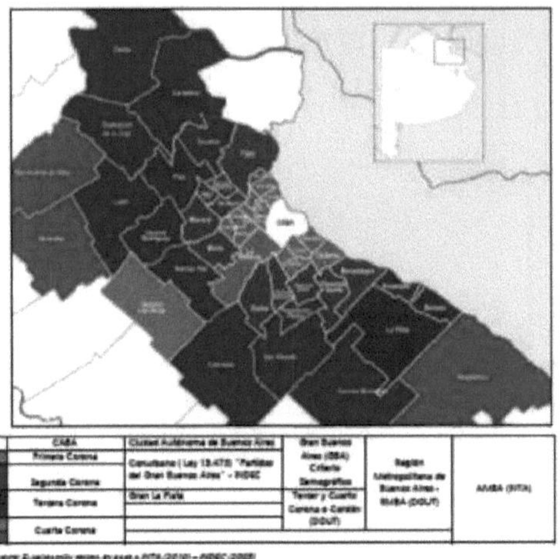

Map 4: Four crowns or cordons surrounding CABA and their location in Buenos Aires Province *(Kozel, A; & col, 2017))*

Donors were classified according to the declared address at the date of donation in 4 categories: CABA, Buenos Aires Province, other provinces and other countries. For the last two categories, the number of donors was marginal both for the total number of donors studied (0.59%) and for those positive for the different TTIs, as can be seen in graphs 29 to 36.

Although the hospital is located in CABA, it receives more donations from inhabitants of the Province of Buenos Aires (55.03%) than from the city itself (44.37%). Similar proportions are seen in positives for Syphilis, Chagas and HCV but not for the other infections studied.

In order to try to better understand the differences in distribution by declared address, a separate analysis has been made for each of these two broad categories.

Donantes según domicilio (2006-2017) N=44244

Gráfico 29: Distribución de los donantes estudiados de acuerdo con su domicilio declarado

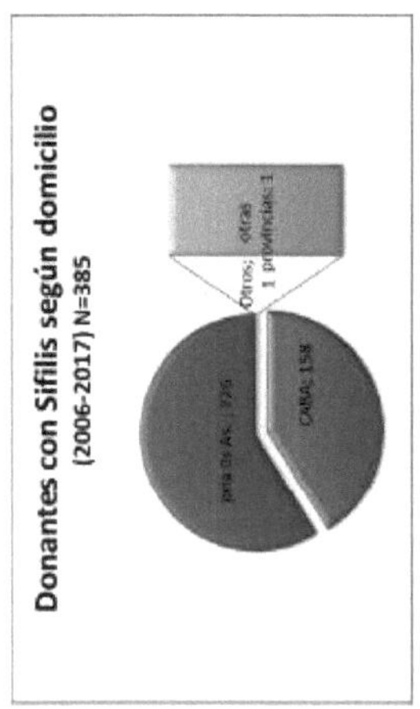

Gráfico 30: Distribución de los donantes con Sífilis de acuerdo con su domicilio declarado

Donantes con Chagas según domicilio (2006-2017) N=713

Gráfico 32: Distribución de los donantes con Chagas de acuerdo con su domicilio declarado.

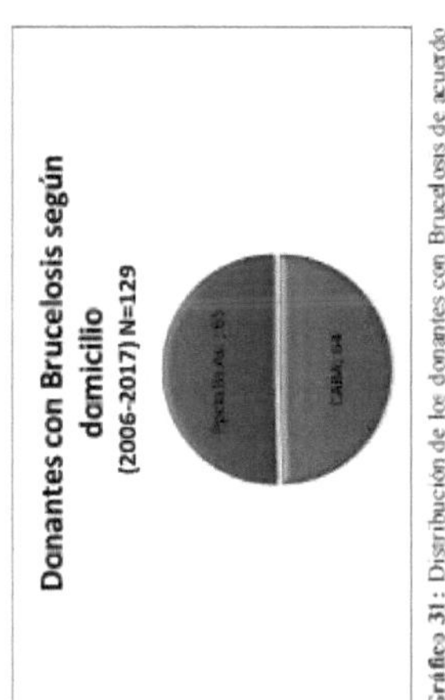

Gráfico 31: Distribución de los donantes con Brucelosis de acuerdo con su domicilio declarado.

Figure 29: Distribution of donors surveyed according to their declared address
Figure 31: Distribution of donors with Brucellosis according to their declared address.
Figure 30: Distribution of donors with Syphilis according to their declared address.
Figure 32: Distribution of donors with Chagas disease according to their declared address.

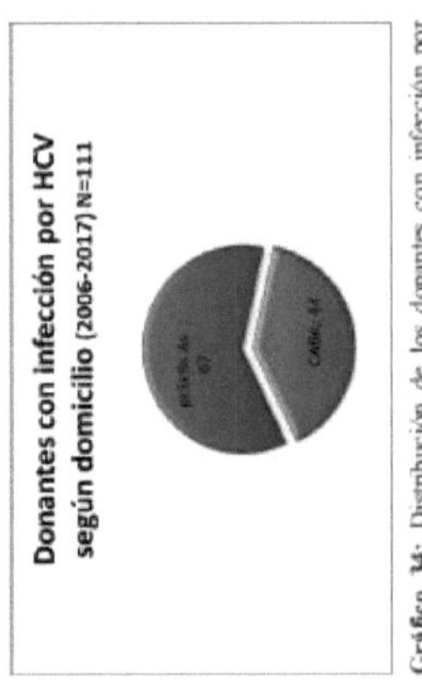

Gráfico 34: Distribución de los donantes con infección por HCV de acuerdo con su domicilio declarado.

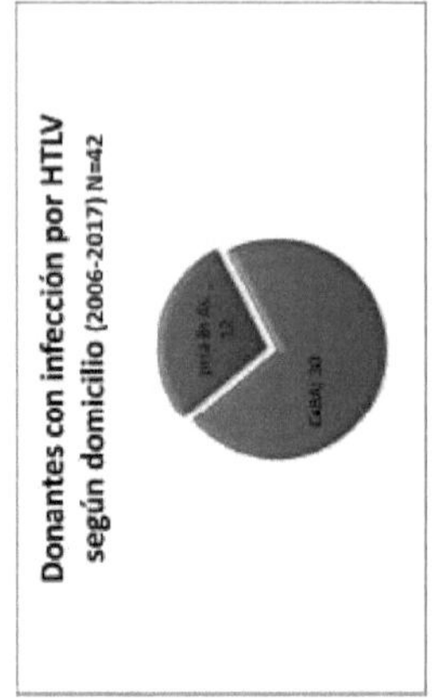

Gráfico 36: Distribución de los donantes con infección por HTLV de acuerdo con su domicilio declarado

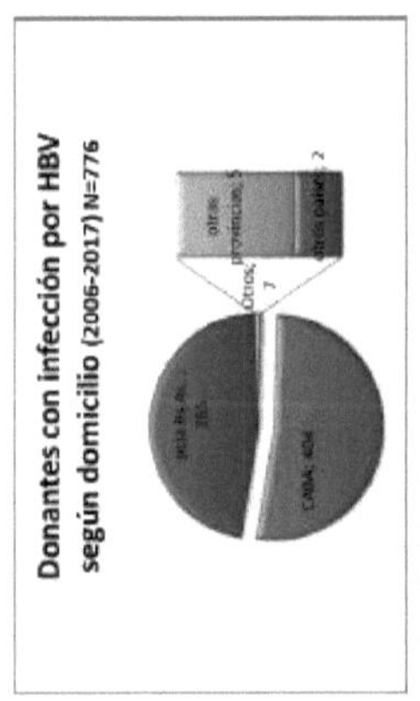

Gráfico 33: Distribución de los donantes con infección por HBV de acuerdo con su domicilio declarado.

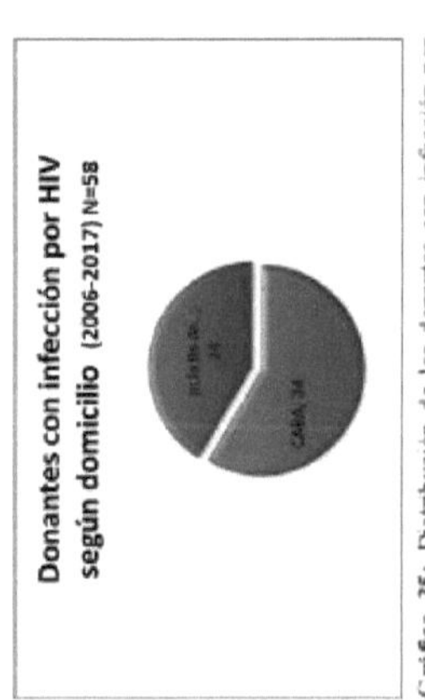

Gráfico 35: Distribución de los donantes con infección por HIV de acuerdo con su domicilio declarado.

Figure 33: Distribution of donors with HBV infection according to their declared address.
Figure 35: Distribution of donors with HIV infection according to their declared address.
Figure 34: Distribution of donors with HCV infection according to their declared address.
Figure 36: Distribution of HTLV-infected donors according to their declared domicile

1. Donors domiciled in CABA

Figure 37 shows the distribution of donors according to each of the 15 communes into which CABA is divided. As can be seen, the largest bar portions, in most of the columns, correspond to communes 1 and 14. The portion corresponding to the other commune that integrates the programme area of the Hospital is not so noticeable: commune 2.

Exceptions to the above are:

- HTLV: in the 14th it is non-existent, but in its place the commune 5, formed by the neighbourhoods of Almagro and Boedo, becomes relevant,
- Brucellosis: Communes 6 and 8 are more important.
- HIV: the areas corresponding to communes 3, 4, 7 are enlarged.

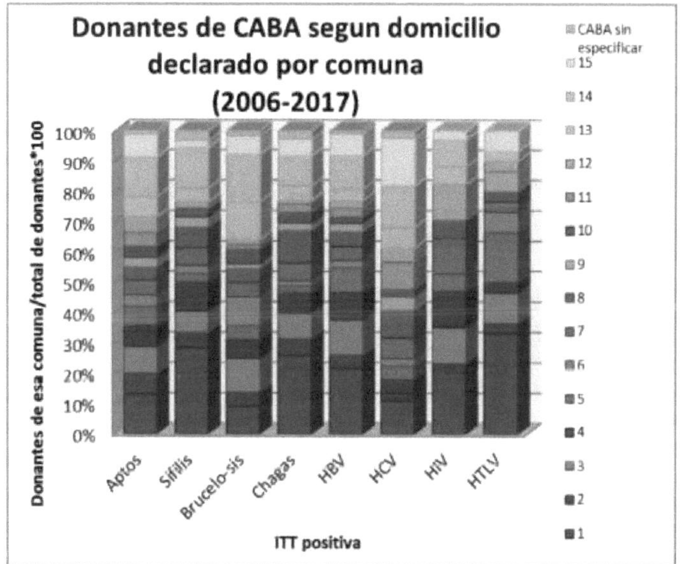

Figure 37: Proportion of donors by commune for the total number of donors domiciled in CABA and for each of the TTIs studied.

If we classify the positive cases for each of the TTIs studied according to commune, the colour that stands out most (graph 38) is that corresponding to HBV infections, followed by Chagas and S^philis, with exceptions such as commune 12 for HIV or commune 11 for HTLV.

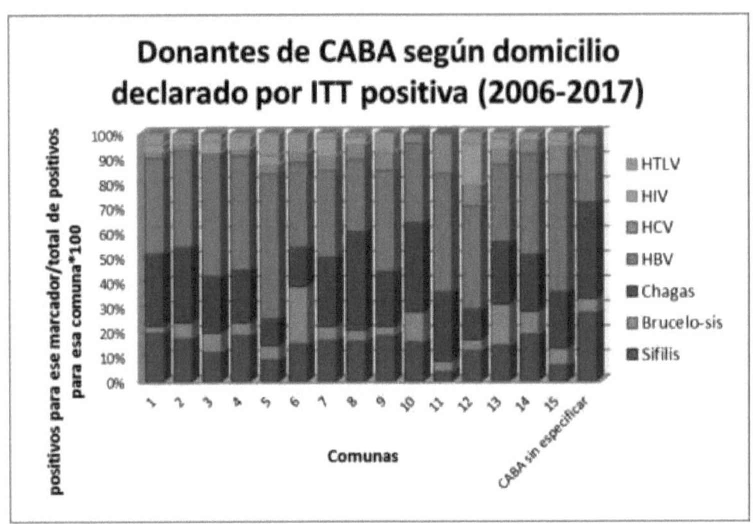

Figure 38: Proportion of donors with positive TTIs by commune

The same is shown in map 5, which shows the geographical relationships of the communes and the total number of donors studied. Similarly, maps 6 to 12 show these relationships by ITT marker. In all of them commune 14 is highlighted, because, as already mentioned, it is the location of the Blood Bank where ëste work was carried out.

Table 13 shows the absolute numbers used to construct these maps. Table 14 shows the distribution of the total number of donors domiciled in CABA, according to commune and place of birth. In this table, special mention is made of the Retiro neighbourhood (commune 1).

Finally, it is important to mention that the percentage of donors born in CABA+Pcia de Bs As, as a percentage of the total of those studied for each commune, ranges from 76.48% (commune 10) to 34.26% in commune 1, being even lower if we take from the latter only the Retiro neighbourhood (21.79%).

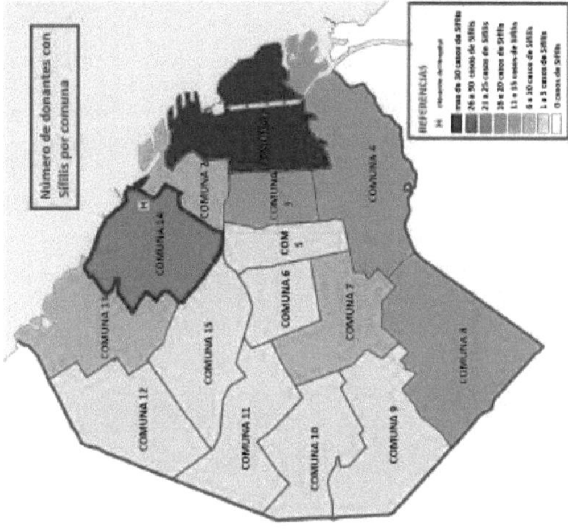

Mapa 6. Donantes con Sífilis según comuna en que se domicilian.

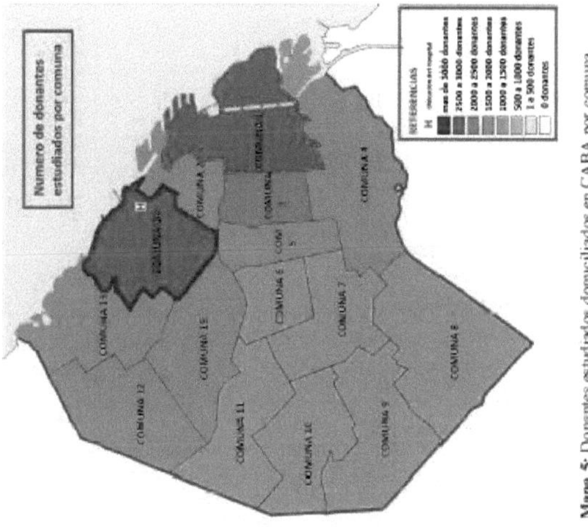

Mapa 5: Donantes estudiados domiciliados en CABA por comuna.

Map 5: Surveyed donors domiciled in CABA by municipality.
Donors with syphilis according to the commune in which they live.

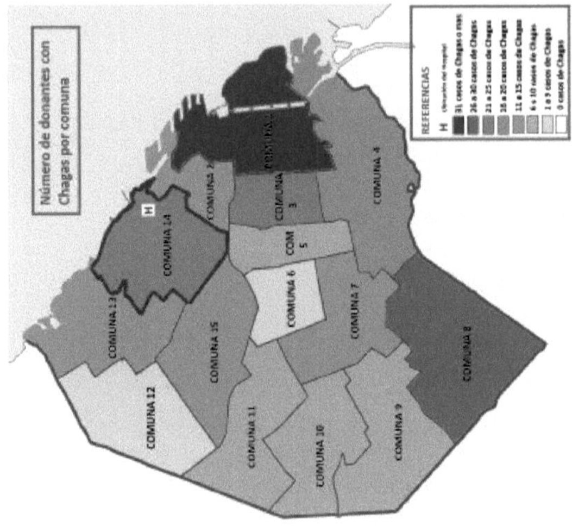

Mapa 8: Donantes con Chagas según comuna en que se domicilian.

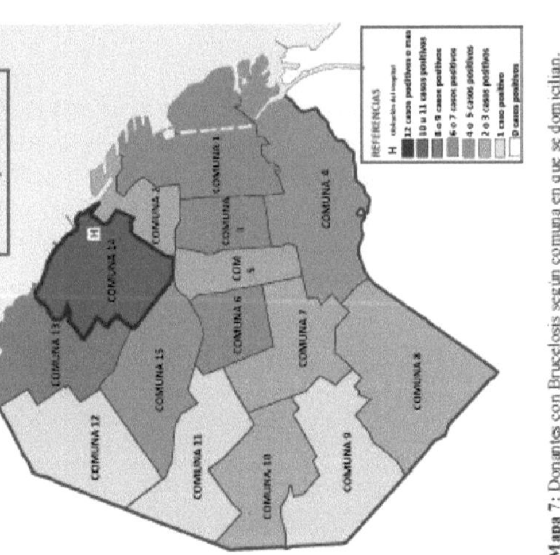

Mapa 7: Donantes con Brucelosis según comuna en que se domicilian.

Mapa 7: Donors with Brucellosis according to the commune in which they were donated.
Map 8: Donors with Chagas disease according to the commune in which they donated.

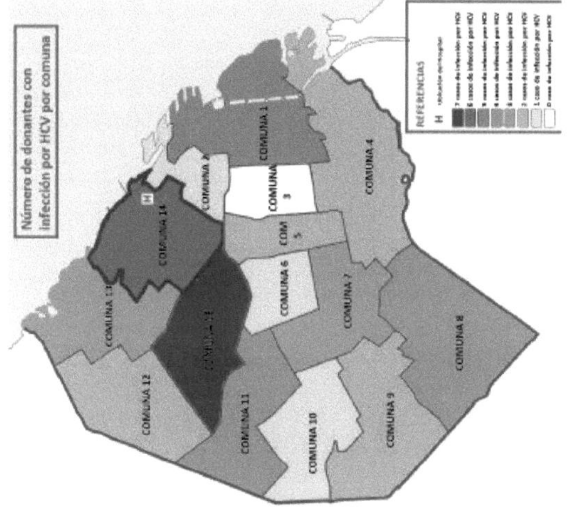

Mapa 10: Donantes con infección por HCV según comuna en que se domicilian.

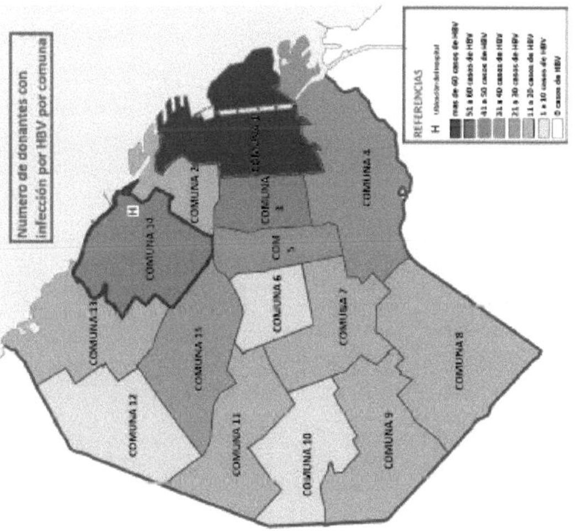

Mapa 3: Donantes con infección por HBV según comuna en que se domicilian

Map 9: Donors with HBV infection by commune of residence.
Mara 10: Donors with HCV infection by commune of residence.

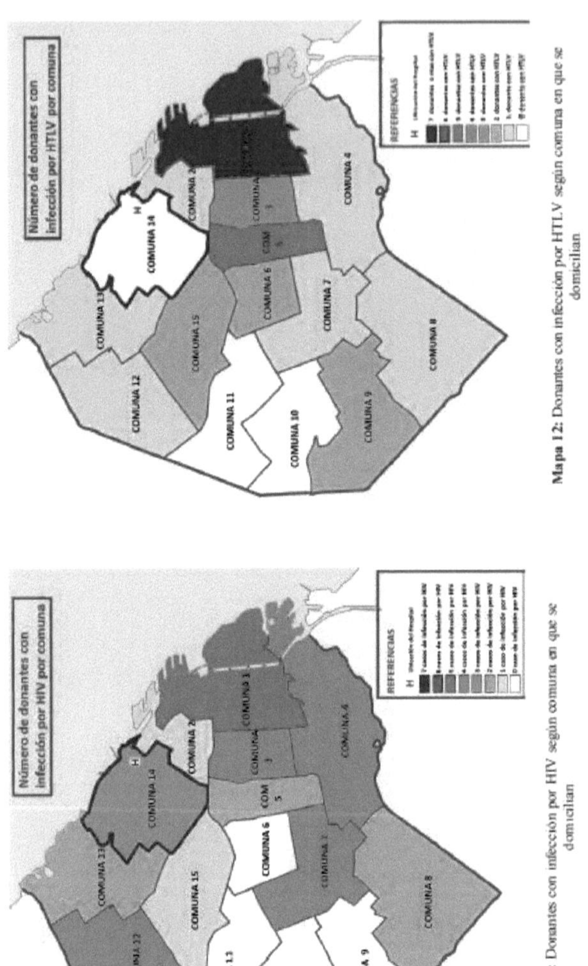

Mara 11: Donors with HIV infection according to the commune in which they were infected.
Mapa 12: Donors with HTLV infection according to the commune in which they were infected.

Commune	Aptos	Syphilis	Brucelosis	Chagas	HBV	HCV	HIV	HTLV
1	2598	45	6	66	88	5	7	10
2	1336	8	3	14	] 18	D 1	1	1
3	1759	. 11	[7]	21	46		4	3
4	1318	15	4	17	Э7	LI 2	4	1
5	1235	5	3	6	□33	]2	2	5
6	755	4	6	4	9	1		2
7	992	9	3	15	' 19	U3	4	1
8	842	[11	3	27	] 20	□	**B2**	1
9	[593	5	1	6	| 11	**E2**		2
10	[710	4	**E3**	9	8	D 1		
11	932	1	1	7	12	L_4		
12	1000	3	1	3	10	U 2	4	D 1
13 "	1308	7	8	12	15	Z3	-r-	-T"
14	**2547**	**21**	**10**	**25**	ZZ4s	**1 6 ~|**	E3	
15	1499	4	"4	14	LI **29**	7	B" 1	2
CABA unspecified	210	5	1	7	4	□ 1		
sum	19634	158	64	253	404	44	34	30

Comuna	Aptos	Sifilis	Brucelosis	Chagas	HBV	HCV	HIV	HTLV
1	2598	45	6	66	88	5	7	10
2	1336	8	3	14	18	1	1	1
3	1759	11	7	21	46		4	3
4	1318	15	4	17	37	2	4	1
5	1235	5	3	6	33	2	2	5
6	755	4	6	4	9	1		2
7	992	9	3	15	19	3	4	1
8	842	11	3	27	20	4	2	1
9	593	5	1	6	11	2		2
10	710	4	3	9	8	1		
11	932	1	1	7	12	4		
12	1000	3	1	3	10	2	4	1
13	1308	7	8	12	15	3	2	1
14	**2547**	**21**	**10**	**25**	**45**	**6**	**3**	
15	1499	4	4	14	29	7	1	2
CABA sin especificar	210	5	1	7	4	1		
suma	19634	158	64	253	404	44	34	30

Table 13: Donors domiciled in CABA, grouped by commune.

CABA		465	393	461	403	437	332	350	297	282	363	429	495	519	841	596	29	6692	Ц-38
CENTRE	GOOD AIR!	425	363	347	249	293	Г232	220	131	128	180	250	E1	406	680	363	15	4553	Ц45
	CORDOBA	18	23	16	10	8	5	13	2	0	10	9	8	16	33	15	0	186	5
	SANTA FE	19	12	20	14	9	10	7	7	8	4	8	14	10	38	18	0	198	7
	ENTRE RIOS	17	31	31	6	12	12	10	0	1	6	11	12	16	49	19	0	233	6
	LA PAMPA	5	7	4	0	0	0	1	1	1	0	2	2	1	5	2	1	32	1
NEA	CURRENTS	41	26	30	22	16	5	9	10	4	5	6	9	20	40	22	7	272	12
	MISSIONS	41	29	36	27	25	8	11	10	6	4	9	8	22	40	22	4	302	14
	CHACO	22	19	14	12	10	5	2	12	8	4	9	10	14	25	10	1	177	8
	FORMOSA	25	10	17	18	13	3	4	2	2	1	1	6	9	15	9	2	137	13
NOA	JUJUY	106	8	37	29	22	3	14	20	4	8	6	4	7	20	9	1	298	1 76
	SALTA	56	20	51	25	22	2	17	14	6	4	5	2	16	30	19	4	293	32
	TUCUMAN	55	16	40	24	19	5	17	6	4	6	10	5	18	34	20	0	279	23
	SANTIAGO DE	41	20	26	18	16	5	15	4	6	6	13	0	7	0	0	1	178	16
	CATAMARCA	6	7	9	5	4	2	2	1	1	1	2	3	4	11	3	0	61	4
	LA RIOJA	2	1	3	0	1	0	2	1	0	0	1	1	2	3	3	0	20	0
CUYO	MENDOZA	25	10	9	6	7	4	2	3	3	4	4	6	6	16	9	0	114	16
	ST JOHN'S	7	6	8	7	8	4	0	1	2	5	1	2	4	13	2	0	70	4
	SAN LUIS	1	5	2	1	5	0	1	0	1	0	2	1	2	3	3	0	27	0
PATAGO-NIA	RIO NEGRO	3	4	4	0	3	1	2	1	0	0	3	1	0	7	1	0	30	0
	NEUQUEN	3	3	5	0	0	1	0	0	1	0	1	1	2	10	2	1	30	0
	SANTA CRUZ	5	3	0	0	4	0	1	1	3	0	0	1	1	4	1	0	24	3
	CHUBUT	3	9	4	1	1	2	1	0	1	1	0	2	8	8	3	0	44	0
	FL LAND	1	2	1	1	0	0	1	0	0	0	1	0	0	1	1	0	9	0
Argentina unspecified		37	22	24	17	19	16	12	8	11	9	10	18	17	81	37	0	338	19
Limitrofes	URUGUAY	19	25	39	23	24	9	7	8	6	8	19	14	17	53	31	1	303	6
	BRAZIL	14	8	17	4	8	1	3	0	0	2	3	1	6	11	7	0	85	3
	PARAGUAY	611	104	115	214	1 69	1 30	78	174	25	25	| 28	1 48	70	210	87	102	1990	|470
	BOLIVIA	172	13	38	57	23	5	98	97	52	30	15	3	8	18	25	20	674	[146
	CHILE	17	12	14	7	11	3	5	2	2	0	2	4	9	13	6	0	107	5
REST OF SOUTH AMERICA	PERU	259	65	279	110	J14	D 38	68	23	21	14	] 58	1 30	49	96	103	20	1347	H12
	COLOMBIA	46	39	19	3	17	8	7	0	0	5	2	3	8	61	11	0	229	10
	ECUADOR	0	0	0	0	0	0	0	0	0	0	1	0	0	1	1	0	3	0
	VENEZUELA	1	1	0	0	0	0	0	0	0	0	0	1	0	0	0	0	3	0
REST OF AMERICA	CUBA	6	3	4	2	1	0	1	0	0	0	1	0	1	8	3	1	31	2
	Rep. DOMINIC	0	1	0	0	0	0	1	1	0	0	0	0	0	0	0	0	3	0
	MEXICO	0	0	0	0	1	0	0	0	0	0	0	0	0	0	0	0	1	0
	USA	1	1	2	0	0	0	0	0	0	0	1	0	3	7	5	0	20	1
EUROPA	GERMANY	5	0	9	0	1	0	1	0	2	1	1	0	2	3	3	0	' 28	0
	AMSTERDAM	2	0	4	1	1	2	0	0	0	0	0	0	0	2	1	0	' 13	0
	SPAIN	6	5	4	1	2	1	1	5	1	1	3	2	4	4	2	0	' 42	1
	FRANCE	4	0	4	0	0	0	0	0	0	2	0	0	0	1	1	0	' 12	0
	GREECE	0	0	0	0	0	0	0	0	0	0	0	0	0	0	1	0	' 1	0
	ITALY	0	0	3	1	2	0	3	0	0	1	2	2	1	6	4	0	' 25	0
	RUSSIA	2	2	1	0	1	0	0	0	0	0	0	0	0	0	1	0	' 7	0
	UKRAINE	2	5	1	0	1	0	1	0	0	0	0	0	0	1	1	0	' 12	0
NEAR EAST	ARMENIA	1	0	0	0	0	0	0	0	0	0	0	0	0	0	0	0	' 1	0
	TURKEY	0	2	1	0	1	0	0	0	0	0	0	0	0	4	0	0	' 8	0
	IRAN	0	0	0	0	0	0	0	0	0	0	0	0	0	1	0	0	' 1	0
	ISRAEL	0	0	0	0	0	0	0	0	0	0	1	0	0	0	0	0	' 1	0
	EGYPT	0	1	0	0	0	0	0	0	0	0	0	0	0	0	0	0	1 1	0
	ALGERIA	0	0	0	0	0	0	0	0	0	0	0	0	0	0	1	0	1 1	0
FAR EAST	JAPAN	0	0	1	0	0	0	0	0	0	0	0	0	0	0	0	0	' 1	1
	TAIWAN	0	0	2	0	0	0	0	0	0	0	0	10	1	38	16	0	' 67	0
	CHINA	1	0	2	0	2	1	2	0	1	0	2	0	2	0	0	0	' 13	0
	KOREA	0	0	1	0	1	0	2	0	0	0	0	0	0	1	0	0	5 5	0
	PHILIPPINES	0	0	0	0	1	0	0	0	0	0	0	0	0	1	0	0	' 2	0
sum		2598	1336	1759	1318	1235	755	992	842	593	710	932	1000	1308	2547	1499	210	19634	1299

Table 14: Total donors domiciled in CABA by commune and place of birth.

ii. Donors domiciled in the Province of Buenos Aires

In graph 39 we can see that around 90% of the donors studied, domiciled in the province of Buenos Aires, live in the GBA. In the ITT positive cases, something similar happens with the Brucellosis exception, where there is a relative increase in the 2nd and 3rd cordon, and for HTLV there is an increase in the interior of the province. Regarding HIV, the proportion of positive cases in the south of GBA is striking.

Donors from the Province of Buenos Aires according to address

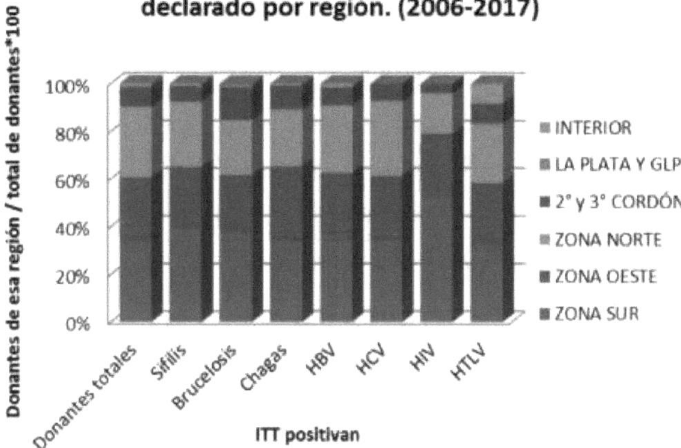

Figure 39: Proportion of donors domiciled in the Province of Buenos Aires by region, for the total and for each of the TTIs studied.

Figure 40 shows the proportion of positive donors for each of the TTIs by region of domicile. Coinciding with the

In the case of CABA, HBV and Chagas infections show the highest proportion of positives in the different regions of the province, followed by syphilis. In Greater La Plata and the interior of the province, the proportions do not follow this pattern. In these cases there may be a distortion due to the small number of donors studied from these regions of the province, as can be seen in the lower part of the table15.

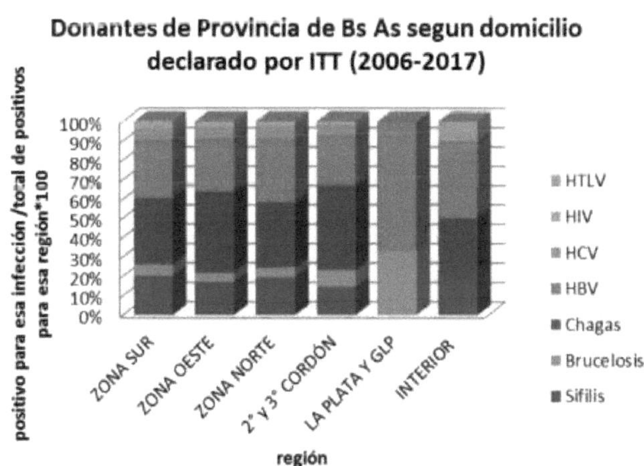

Figure 40: Proportion of TTI positive donors by region of Buenos Aires Province.

REGION	Total donors	Syphilis	Brucellosis	Chagas	HBV	HCV	HIV	HTLV
ZONASUR	8348	90	25	155	135	23	13	4
1° CORDON GBA WEST ZONE	6449	57	15	141	03	10	8	3
NORTH ZONE	7192	62	15	109	104	21	4	3

2nd and 3rd CORDON	1967	15	9	46	27	5	1	1
SILVER AND LPG	142	0	1	0	2	0	0	0
INTERIOR	250	2	0	3	4	0	0	1
Sum	24348	226	65	454	365	67	24	12

Table 15: Donors domiciled in the province of Buenos Aires grouped by geographic area and cordon or corona

Below is the geographic location of donors domiciled in the first cordon of the GBA (map 13) and what happens with the positives for each of the 7 ITIs studied (map 14 to 20).

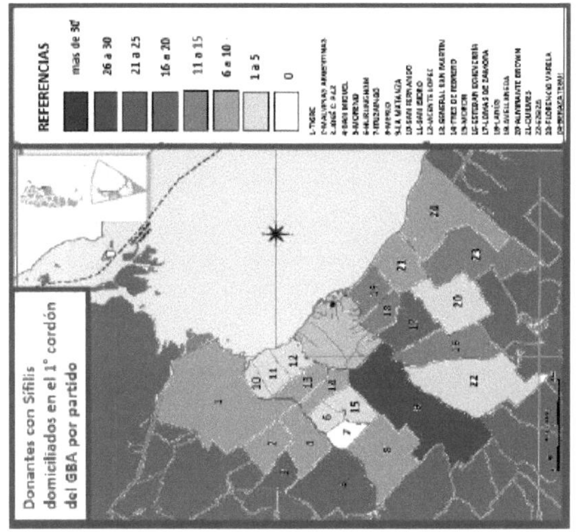

Mapa 14: Donantes con Sífilis según partido del 1° cordón del GBA en el que se domicilian

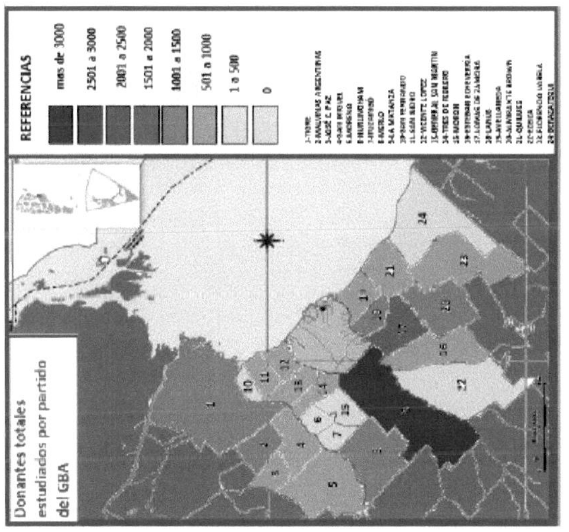

Mapa 13: Donantes estudiados domiciliados en el 1° cordón del GBA por partido.

Mapa 13: Donors studied domiciled in the 1st cordon of the GBA by party.
Mapa 14: Donors with Syphilis according to the match of the 1st cordon of the GBA in which they were infected.

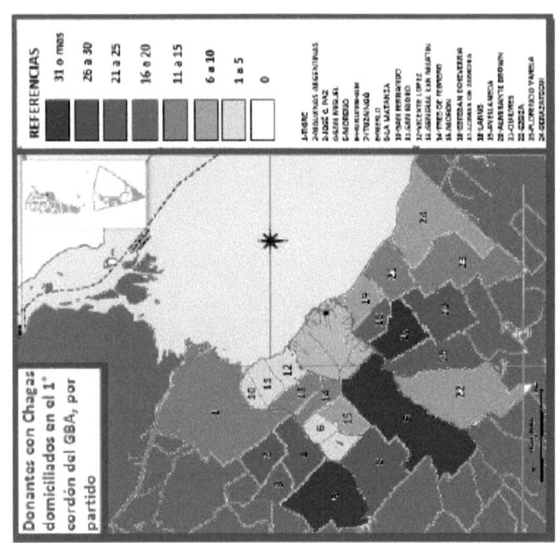

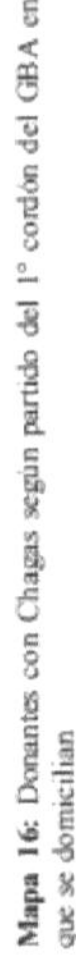
Mapa 16: Donantes con Chagas según partido del 1° cordón del GBA en el que se domicilian

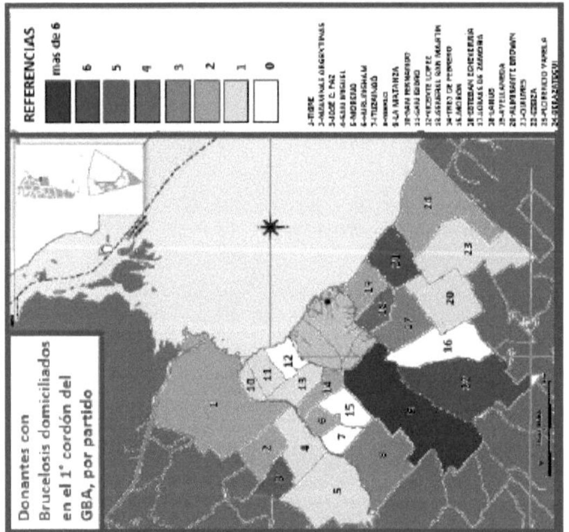

Mapa 15: Donantes con Brucelosis según partido del 1° cordón del GBA en el que se domicilian.

Map 15: Donors with Brucellosis according to the district of the 1st GBA cordon in which they are infected.
Map 16: Donors with Chagas disease according to the district of the first GBA cordon in which they were infected.

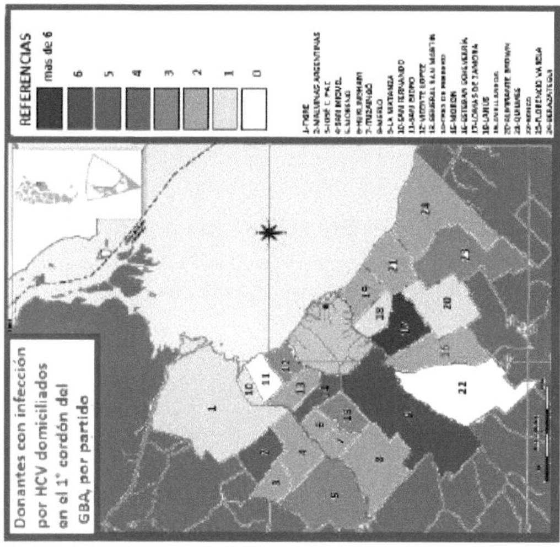

Mapa 18: Donantes con infección por HCV según partido del 1° cordón del GBA en el que se domicilian.

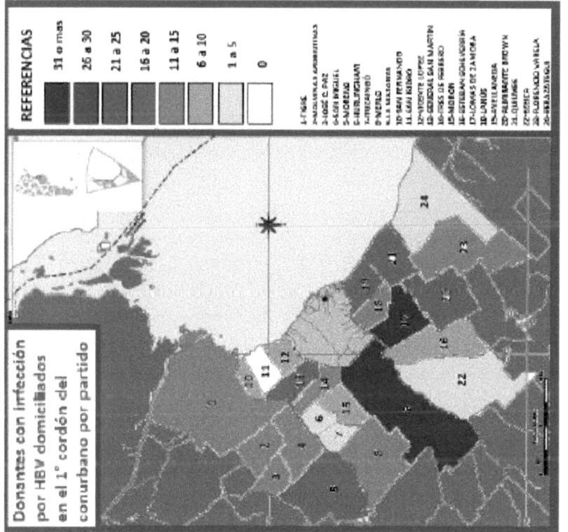

Mapa 17: Donantes con infección por HBV según partido del 1° cordón del GBA en el que se domicilian.

Map 17: Donors with HBV infection according to the district of the 1st GBA cordon in which they are infected.
Mara 18: Donors with HCV infection according to the first GBA district in which they were infected.

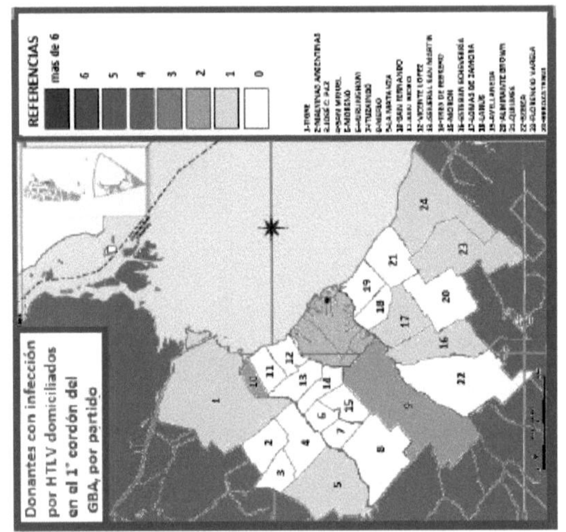

Mapa 20: Donantes con infección por HTLV según partido del 1° cordón del GBA en el que se domicilian.

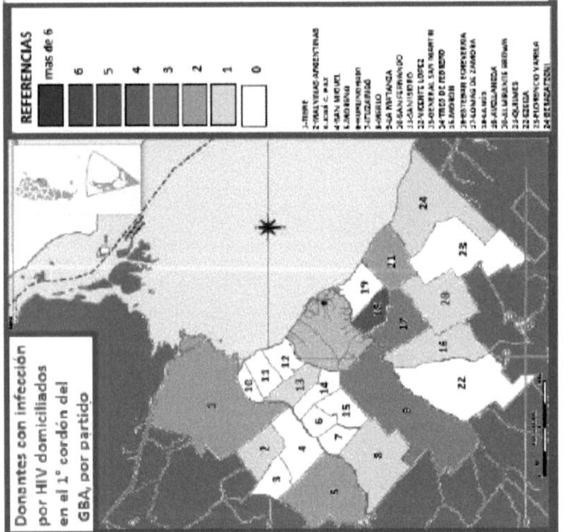

Mapa 19: Donantes con infección por HIV según partido del 1° cordón del GBA en el que se domicilian.

Mapa 19: Donors with HIV infection according to the first district of the GBA in which they are infected.
Mapa 20: Donors with HTLV infection according to the first district of the GBA in which they are infected.

Región	Provincia	partido del GBA																							
		Tigre	Malvinas Arg	J. C. Paz	San Miguel	Moreno	HurlingAM	Ituzaingo	Merlo	La Matanza	San Fernando	San Isidro	V. Lopez	San Martin	3 de Febrero	Moron	E Echeverria	Lomas de Zamora	Lanus	Avellaneda	A Brown	Quilmes	Ezeiza	F. Varela	Berazategui	total
CABA		358	157	119	148	374	101	94	285	1047	62	128	282	197	294	151	156	410	331	198	211	158	89	102	80	5127
	BUENOS AIR	564	627	401	342	429	152	150	472	1079	196	274	321	392	350	221	303	682	428	419	558	501	181	380	309	9691
CENTRO	CORDOBA	5	9	4	5	5	5	5	11	16	5	1	2	11	8	8	6	7	7	10	6	7	1	3	4	151
	SANTA FE	10	2	5	4	2	5	2	7	15	5	3	3	9	5	1	5	12	11	8	11	7	3	5	14	158
	ENTRE RIOS	16	24	1	15	11	9	2	12	34	5	0	7	7	10	4	3	16	10	7	11	6	4	8	7	235
	LA PAMPA	0	0	0	1	0	0	0	1	2	0	1	0	0	0	0	0	0	1	2	2	1	1	0	2	14
NEA	CORRIENTES	18	24	25	19	18	11	4	19	36	5	6	8	13	24	11	19	29	20	14	25	21	5	26	8	408
	MISIONES	12	20	14	24	19	3	4	31	61	6	6	2	14	13	3	14	26	14	13	18	9	12	12	6	356
	CHACO	16	32	27	19	40	3	4	24	45	13	14	6	14	11	7	17	42	28	18	25	21	12	20	13	471
	FORMOSA	10	7	7	8	12	4	2	8	22	1	5	2	6	4	0	11	16	22	3	9	12	7	12	4	194
NOA	JUJUY	6	7	5	4	1	1	1	10	29	1	2	3	7	4	2	8	15	7	16	5	8	3	3	8	156
	SALTA	6	9	7	9	9	3	1	17	24	3	2	5	9	10	2	3	11	12	6	17	10	6	5	6	192
	TUCUMAN	10	30	14	15	15	8	3	28	61	7	6	6	14	12	4	8	16	20	14	18	15	5	11	11	351
	SANTIAGO D	15	38	36	20	32	9	6	32	80	2	3	4	12	12	5	7	40	28	8	33	12	7	17	6	462
	CATAMARCA	3	7	1	3	3	0	1	3	11	3	2	1	3	2	0	0	5	3	0	3	1	3	1	2	61
	LA RIOJA	2	2	1	1	0	0	0	3	3	1	2	1	1	2	1	0	2	2	1	1	1	0	0	0	27
CUYO	MENDOZA	1	8	5	3	5	0	0	3	9	0	1	2	4	7	2	4	6	7	5	1	3	2	5	5	88
	SAN JUAN	3	5	3	1	3	3	0	3	4	0	0	3	1	3	1	0	4	5	3	1	1	0	1	1	49
	SAN LUIS	0	3	6	2	2	1	3	2	2	0	0	2	1	1	2	3	0	2	1	2	2	0	0	0	37
PATAGO-NIA	RIO NEGRO	1	2	0	1	1	0	0	0	0	0	1	2	0	0	0	0	1	1	1	1	1	0	0	0	13
	NEUQUEN	0	1	0	0	1	1	0	0	3	1	0	1	0	0	0	1	2	1	1	1	0	0	0	0	14
	SANTA CRUZ	0	0	0	0	0	0	0	1	2	1	1	0	0	0	0	0	0	0	0	1	1	1	0	0	8
	CHUBUT	0	0	0	0	1	0	1	1	3	0	0	3	0	0	0	0	1	1	1	1	1	0	0	0	14
	TIERRA DEL F	0	0	0	0	0	0	0	0	0	0	0	0	0	0	0	0	0	0	0	1	0	0	0	0	1
Argentina sin especificar		16	20	11	9	14	3	6	18	42	3	6	13	11	11	7	8	30	21	18	15	11	4	11	9	317
Limítrofes	URUGUAY	16	5	4	10	9	2	4	7	16	1	6	9	8	13	7	6	7	13	15	3	4	3	6	2	176
	BRASIL	3	0	1	1	0	1	2	1	2	2	1	3	3	1	0	1	2	4	0	0	2	0	0	1	31
	PARAGUAY	94	49	68	111	146	26	7	89	489	41	27	21	88	64	12	143	286	125	94	120	160	59	109	26	2414
	BOLIVIA	11	4	2	3	16	2	4	13	100	1	1	2	3	9	3	7	34	9	4	3	6	2	7	15	261
	CHILE	2	0	1	2	5	1	2	1	7	2	0	6	2	4	1	7	5	4	6	3	2	2	0	1	66
RESTO SUDAMERICA	PERU	16	3	3	3	10	3	2	9	27	29	20	23	33	22	3	5	30	23	49	9	4	8	2	4	340
	COLOMBIA	1	1	1	1	0	1	0	0	8	0	2	3	1	0	0	0	2	1	0	0	1	0	0	1	24
RESTO AMERICA	CUBA	0	1	0	0	0	0	0	0	0	0	1	4	0	0	0	0	0	1	0	0	0	0	0	0	7
	CANADA	0	0	0	0	0	0	0	0	0	0	0	0	0	0	0	1	0	0	0	0	0	0	0	0	1
	USA	0	1	0	0	0	0	0	0	1	3	0	0	0	0	0	0	0	0	0	1	0	0	0	0	6
EUROPA	ALEMANIA	0	0	0	0	0	0	0	0	2	1	2	0	2	1	0	1	1	1	1	0	0	0	0	0	12
	SUIZA	0	0	0	0	1	0	0	0	0	0	0	0	0	0	0	0	0	0	0	0	0	0	0	0	1
	AMSTERDAM	0	0	0	0	0	0	0	0	0	0	0	0	0	1	0	0	0	0	0	0	0	0	0	1	2
	ESPAÑA	1	0	0	2	2	0	1	1	2	0	1	0	0	0	2	2	1	0	1	1	1	0	0	0	18
	FRANCIA	0	0	0	0	0	0	0	0	0	0	0	1	0	0	0	0	0	0	0	0	0	0	0	0	1
	GRECIA	0	0	0	0	0	1	0	0	0	0	0	0	0	0	0	0	0	0	0	0	0	0	0	0	1
	ITALIA	0	0	0	0	2	1	1	1	3	0	0	1	4	1	2	0	0	1	1	1	1	0	0	0	20
	RUSIA	0	0	0	0	0	0	0	0	1	0	0	1	0	0	1	0	0	0	0	0	0	0	0	0	3
	UCRANIA	0	1	0	0	0	0	0	0	0	0	0	0	0	1	0	0	0	1	1	1	0	0	0	0	5
LEJANO ORIENTE	TAIWAN	0	0	0	0	0	0	0	0	0	0	0	1	0	0	1	0	0	0	0	0	0	0	0	0	2
	COREA	0	0	0	1	0	0	0	1	1	0	0	0	0	0	0	0	0	0	0	0	0	0	0	0	3
suma		1016	1099	790	787	988	360	314	1074	3249	400	571	759	870	900	464	749	1740	1218	939	1119	991	400	746	446	21989

Table 16: Total number of donors in the Province of Buenos Aires according to district and place of birth.

CHAPTER 5

13) Co-infections

Graph 41 shows that the most frequent co-infection in the donors studied is Chagas disease with HBV infection, followed by Syphilis with HBV infection, and in third place is simultaneous infection with both hepatitis B and C. Table 17 complements the data in the above-mentioned table by describing the less frequent co-infections, including co-infections involving three of the micro-organisms studied.

Adding cases together, 77.32% of co-infections involved HBV and 56.7% involved Chagas disease.

Most frequent co-infections in

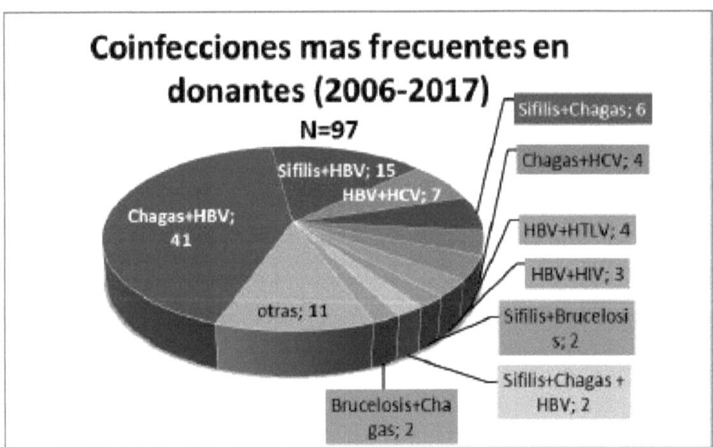

Figure 41: Co-infections in donors studied (2006-2017)

other co-infections	N
syphilis+HBV+HIV	1
syphilis+HCV	1
syphilis+HIV	1
syphilis+HTLV	1
brucellosis+HBV	1
brucellosis+HBV+HIV	1
brucellosis+HCV	1
chagas+HBV+HCV	1
HCV+HIV	1
HCV+HTLV	1
HIV+HTLV	1

Table 17 : Co-low frequency infections in donors (2006-2017)

The co-infections can be seen in the following graphs that occurred with each of the 7 TTIs studied, with the least co-infections being Brucellosis and HTLV infection, followed by HIV.

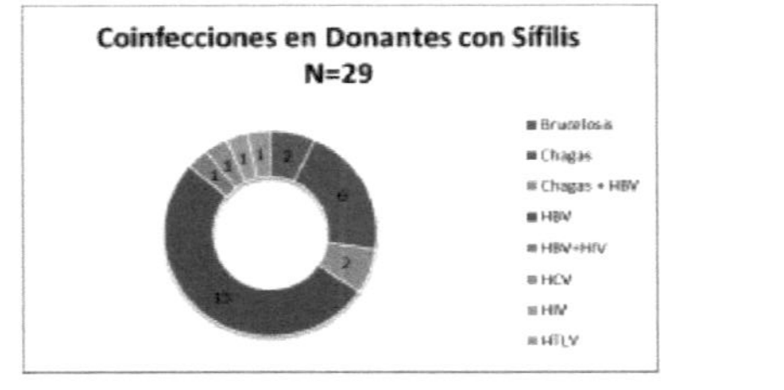

Gráfico 42: Distribución de las co-infecciones en donantes con Sífilis (2006-2017)

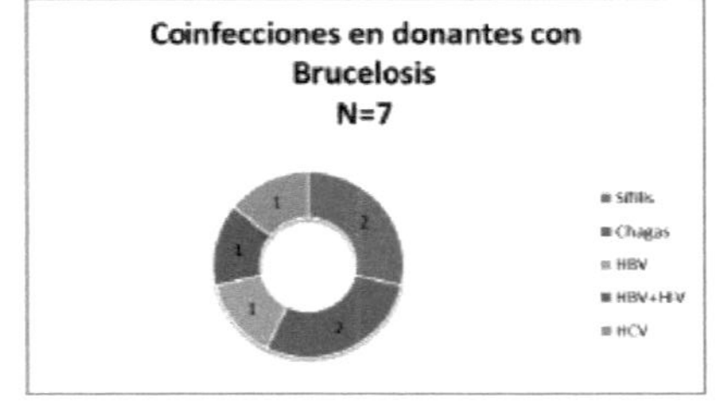

Gráfico 43: Distribución de las co-infecciones en donantes con Brucelosis (2006-2017).

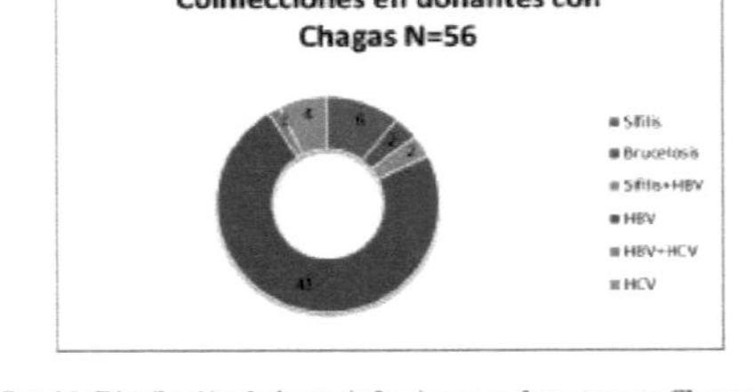

Gráfico 44: Distribución de las co-infecciones en donantes con Chagas (2006-2017)

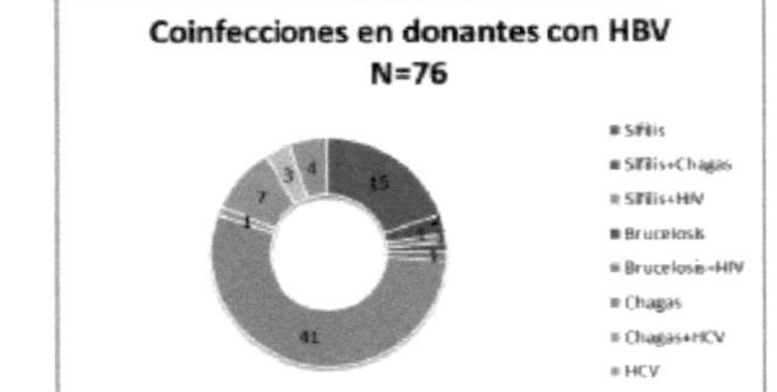

Gráfico 45: Distribución de las co-infecciones en donantes con infección por HBV (2006-2017).

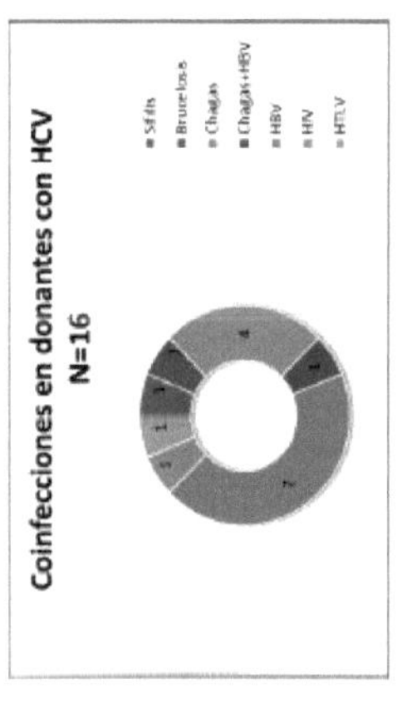

Gráfico 46: Distribución de las co-infecciones en donantes con infección por HCV (2006-2017)

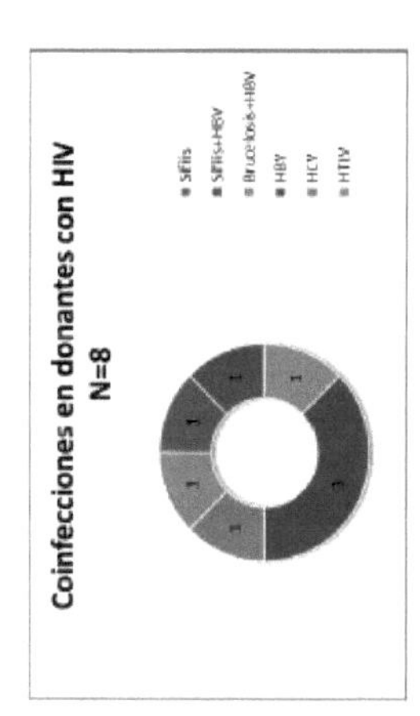

Gráfico 47: Distribución de las co-infecciones en donantes con infección por HIV (2006-2017)

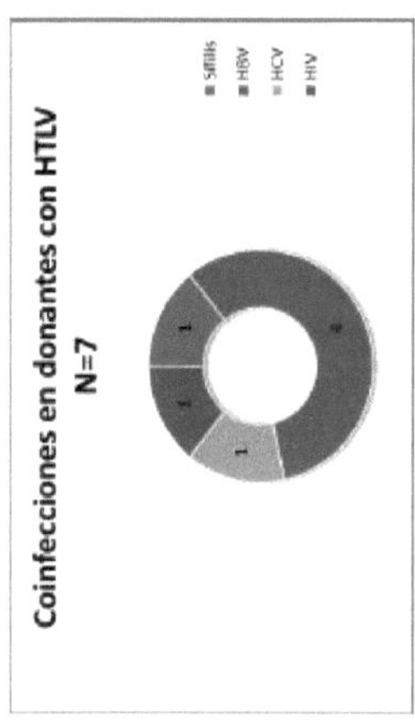

Gráfico 48: Distribución de las co-infecciones en donantes con infección por HTLV (2006-2017)

Figure 42: Distribution of co-infections in donors with Syphilis (2006- 2017)
Figure 43: Distribution of co-infections in donors with Brucellosis (2006-2017).
Figure 44: Distribution of co-infections in donors with Chagas disease (2006- 2017)
Figure 45: Distribution of co-infections in donors with HBV infection (2006-2017).
Figure 46: Distribution of co-infections in HCV-infected donors (2006-2017)
Figure 47: Distribution of co-infections in HIV-infected donors (2006-2017)
Figure 48: Distribution of co-infections in donors with HTLV infection (2006-2017)

CHAPTER 6

14) Discussion

Those who approach the Intrahospital Blood Banks to find out about the conditions to be accepted as a donor are given explanations similar to those given in voluntary blood donation campaigns, campaigns that are carried out in private companies, public roads, etc. These campaigns *(Laplagne & col, 2015)* explain, among other concepts, the requirements to qualify as a donor. Therefore, if the person, sensitised by these campaigns or by the information received in the BSI, perceives themselves as healthy, they donate. And many of them do so repeatedly, becoming altruistic voluntary donors. On the other hand, those who, thanks to these campaigns, learn that some condition they suffer from is a reason for rejection in the medical-clinical interview, automatically refrain from presenting themselves as voluntary donors. It is therefore natural that deferral is lower in this group *(Gendler & Trinca, 2013)*, as shown in numerous studies.

For all these reasons, one would expect that only those who are healthy would donate blood. However, this is not always the case. Therefore, in the medical-clinical interview there are specific questions to detect the "unhealthy" and to defer them, temporarily or permanently, depending on the reason for the deferral *(Plan Nac. de Sasngre, Min. de Salud, sf)*.

Of the total number of admissions to the Donor Book in the period 2006-2017, only 62.41% were eligible for this study, and the total percentage of donors deferred during the medical-clinical interview was 21.94%, with a minimum of 2.5% and a maximum of 42.47% depending on the year). This total percentage is close to that reported by other CABA hospitals *(Borgareto & col, 2015; Gama & col, 2018)*, lower than that of the Htal.

Paroissien de I. Casanova, partido de La Matanza *(Osatnik & Matsuya, 2013)* and larger than in collections *(Martin & col, 2017)*.

These differences in the percentage of deferral could be related to the socio-economic conditions of the donor and/or his self-perception of his health status. The socio-economic conditions of the districts in which the Blood Banks are located, measured as NBI, in our case are not sufficient to explain the difference in the percentage of deferred donors, since the levels of this index for La Matanza (*Dir. Prov. de Estad., Min. de Economda, Pcia. As; Quesada Aramburu, J & col, 2012)* are similar to those of commune 4 *(Dir. Gral. de Estad. y Censos, GCBA, 2010)* commune in which the hospital cited by Borgareto *(2015)* is located, Consequently, to explain the level of deferral it would be necessary to delve deeper into the issue of self-perception of health status. The number of units ordered from the network (table 8, column of units studied in other centres) fluctuates, with some peaks in demand, such as in 2013, when, due to a decrease in the supply from our own donors, we had to resort to the network to meet the hospital's internal demand.

Table 9 and Graph 3 show that the greatest number of positive results in the Blood Bank are due to HBV infections and secondly to Chagas disease. Already in 2012, in a multicentre study *(Gendler & col, 2011)* on the discarding of units by reactive serology, it was stated that the main causes of discarding were these two infections, with seroreactivity for Chagas of 3.25% (SD.7%) and for HBcAc of 2.71 (SD.34). At this point it should be clarified that these RRs include all positives, whether true or false. For this reason, it cannot be affirmed that, with respect to the 2012 study, there has been an inversion of proportions or an increase in HBV (which is not shown in Graph 7) or that there has simply been a decrease in Chagas, despite the fact that Graph 6 shows a downward trend, in line with the decrease in acute cases of Chagas that can be seen in the successive Epidemiological Bulletins of the National Ministry of Health *(Min. of Health, Argentina, n.d.).*

However, if we compare the results obtained here with those shown in the Boletin Epidemiologico n°458 (*Varela, & col, 2019)* on page 39, we see a difference with our results: there, the positive cases of Chagas disease reported are in first place while Hepatitis B is in last place because they only took HBsAg into account for their report and not other markers for this infection (such as HBcAc, which is included here). What this study does agree with this bulletin is the decrease in the number of cases of Chagas disease.

In third and fourth place among the Blood Bank positives are bacterial infections: Syphilis and Brucellosis (Graph 3), which in the annual prevalence study show a large fluctuation in the percentages for the former, with a maximum in 2015 and an increase for the latter (Graphs 4 and 5 respectively).

Lastly, HCV, HIV and HTLV viral infections are the minority but no less important due to their morbimortality (hepatocarcinoma, cirrhosis, for the first *(Angeleri & col 2016)*, recurrent and/or opportunistic infections with depletion of the immune system for the second *(OPS/WHO, 2009)* and degenerative neurological or oncohematological problems for the third *(ColuccI & col, 2016)) and due to the consequences for those around these infected persons due to the precautions they must take to avoid becoming infected or the care they must take when they are no longer asymptomatic. col s, 2016))* and the consequences for those around these infected people because of the precautions they must take to avoid becoming infected or the care they must provide for these people when they are no longer asymptomatic.

Turning to the fluctuations in the annual prevalence of S^filis, this is at odds with what is reported in the integrated epidemiological bulletin n°458 *(Varela& col, 2019)* which states that "the percentage of positive samples is decreasing until 2015 and has remained relatively stable since then". In contrast, in ëste Centro there was a progressive increase between 2009 and 2015. This difference in behaviour may be reflecting the fact that ëste particular boletm graphs the total pa^s of complaints for Blood Bank and does not make the breakdown by province, knowing that each one has very different realities.

But if we analyse previous bulletins *(Secr. de Promotion y Programas Sanitarios, Min. de Salud, Argentina, 2012; Secr. de Promotion y Programas Sanitarios, Min. de Salud, Argentina, 2013; Secr.de Promocion y Programas Sanitarios, Min. de Salud, Argentina, 2014; Antman J & col, 2015; Antman J & col, 2016; Echenique A & col, 2017; Secr. de Promocion y Programas Sanitarios, Min. de Salud, Argentina, 2018)* we see that there was a decrease in reported cases of early and unspecified S^philis between 2007 and 2010 and then a gradual rise in the central region of the country, the region to which CABA belongs, and consequently ëste Bank.

In the population studied there was a gradual increase in the prevalence of Brucellosis (graph 5). In this case there is also no concordance with the results reported in the epidemiological bulletin 485 at the national level.

Figure 8 shows that the 'annual prevalence of HCV is lower at the end of the period than at the beginning of the period, a theme to which we will return later.

With regard to the gender distribution of donors, the low proportion of female donors compared to the general population is striking (Table 11 and Figure 13). Although deferred donors were not the subject of this study, the population pyramid for this group was constructed to represent the findings (Figure 12). This graph shows that the number of men and women deferred is similar, as also shown in the work of E Gonzalez et al *(2017)*.

As the number of women is slightly higher than that of men in the general population (graph 11), a simple mathematical exercise suggests that women are less likely to present themselves as blood donors, in line with *Rossi & Godoy (Rossi & Godoy, 2017)*. Gomes R *(2007)* explained this by suggesting that women consult health services more than men and therefore know more about their pathologies and therefore exclude themselves from donation, in line with what has already been said about self-perception.

Regardless of the causes, which are not the subject of the study, the predominance of men over women (1.58 men for every woman) in the donor population can be seen. This is also true for the positives of the different infections (graphs 14 to 20), with some variations, such as in Brucellosis (graph 15) where the difference is the smallest (1.39 men for every woman) or in HIV (graph 19) where it is greater. In contrast to our experience, there are Latin American studies that show a higher prevalence of Brucellosis in women than in men *(Mndez-Lozano, Rodnguez-Reyes, & Sanchez-Zamorano, 2015; Oliveira Cavalcanti Soares & col, 2015)* and relate this to the higher proportion of women attending health check-ups, but these studies have not been conducted in the Blood Donor population. Conversely, men who are aware of their work-related condition (or suspect it) may exclude themselves as donors.

As already mentioned, in the case of HIV (Figure 19), the proportion of men among the positives is much higher than that of women (3.8 men/women). This exceeds that described by the HIV-AIDS Bulletin for the general population *(Direction de Sida, ETS, Hepatitis and TBC, 2018)*, according to which the rate of diagnoses in men is twice that of women.

As one of the requirements to donate blood is to be of legal age (or to have the permission of a parent or guardian if not), the lowest quintile in graphs 11 to 20 is the one that includes those between 15 and 19 years of age. This quintile is particularly small in terms of the number of donors, as 15, 16 and 17 year olds very rarely donate blood. Therefore, the analysis should be directed to the next quintile.

Another requirement to donate is to be healthy. As the growth/ageing of people goes hand in hand with the onset of disease and physical deterioration, the older the age, the fewer "healthy" people are available to donate blood or platelets. Figure 13 shows that, after an initial increase in the number of donors in the younger age groups, a peak is reached in the 25-29 age group. Then, as age increases, the number of donors decreases, in both sexes, coinciding with that reported by other centres in CABA *(Gartia & col, 2018)*.

But when we turn to the positive donors for each of the different TTIs, we see that the age distribution is different for each case. The age and sex distribution for S^philis cases (Figure 14) most closely resembles that of the total donors. But the resemblance is not total as the decrease in the number of cases is "delayed" leading to a higher number of infections in the fertility stage in women. This brings risks to her offspring and herself *(WHO, 2015)*. This delay is observed in both sexes.

Something similar is seen in Brucellosis (graph 15), where the decrease in cases for women occurs from the age of 45 years onwards.

For HBV (graph 17) the decrease in the number of cases occurs only after the age of 50, when the total number of donors is also very low. This shows a presence of HBV in the whole population without distinction of specific age groups.

As only 15-20% of hepatitis C virus hepatitis C cases show symptoms in the acute stage, the rest remain asymptomatic for many years *(Webster et al, 2015)* and develop into chronic hepatitis. Therefore, many carriers of this virus learn of their condition as a result of an act of generosity: donating blood. Today, with biosecurity measures in place, infection is much lower and rarely occurs in the health care setting. This is consistent with the slight decrease in average annual prevalence discussed above (graph 8) and with the image in graph 18. The latter shows that in men the frequency of cases increases with age, showing a peak in the 35-39 age group, then decreases and increases again in the over-45 age group.

This report indicates that more than half of the cases reported are due to infection during surgery or through transfusions. This may be related to a late incorporation, in our environment, of the use of biosecurity measures *(Alter, MJ; & col, 1998; Centers for Disease Control and Prevention, 1999; Barril & Traver, 2003)*, including serological screening. In our Bank, the anti-HCV reaction was added to the serological routine in the mid-1990s *(Gendler S., 2005)*.

However, contrary to what Vladimirsky et al *(2015)* described, it can be seen in graph 18 that, in the group of young women (20-29 years), the number of HCV positives is higher than in the other age groups.

For Chagas disease (graph 16) the age distribution shows bars of similar magnitude between 20 and 54 years for women, but for men between 30 and 39 years there is an increase. Something similar occurs for HTLV (graph 20). While for HIV, the increase occurs at slightly higher ages (graph 19).

When analysing the place of birth of the total donors included in the study, we see that more than 65% of them are from the central region, a region that includes CABA and the province of Buenos Aires. CABA is shown separately in Figures 22 to 29 to highlight that most of the donors are not born in the jurisdiction where the study was conducted, so any Public Health intervention to reduce the cases of these infections should be done in coordination with the other geographic areas.

Figure 21 shows that the proportion of donors who were not born in Argentina is 19.62%. Among these there were 8441 born in the American continent of which 6371 are from neighbouring countries, mainly Paraguay and Bolivia (see table 12). Several of the infections investigated are endemic in different parts of the Americas. Migrations from these places contribute to increase the number of positive cases in our donors. The best example can be seen in HTLV (Figure 28) where those born outside Argentina, in countries with endëmic areas for this virus (Takatani & col, 2017; Romani, 2010; Cooper & col, 2009) account for 59.52% of positive cases.

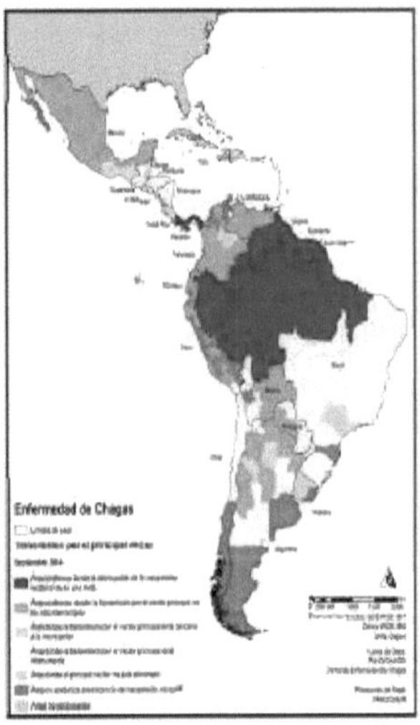

Map 21: Risk of vector-borne transmission of Chagas disease (PHAO/CHA/CD/Control de enfermedad de Chagas, 2014)

Following the same reasoning (see table 12) we have the case of Chagas disease in donors born in Paraguay and Bolivia (see map 21). Something similar occurs with HBV in donors born in Peru and Paraguay (see map 22), countries with a higher prevalence than Argentina according to WHO. A similar phenomenon also occurs with S^philis in the Paraguayan community in Argentina.

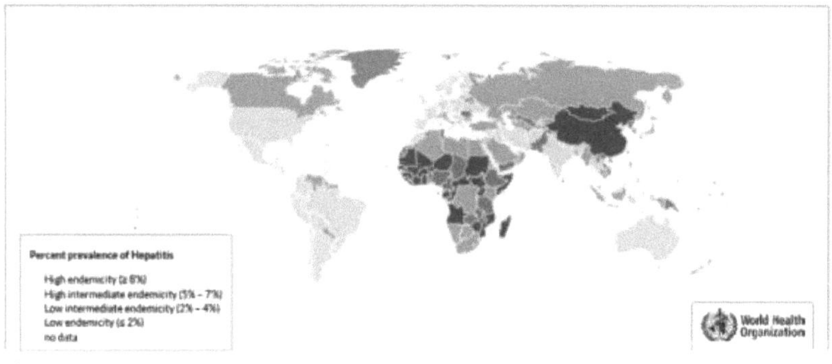

Map 22: Prevalence of HBsAg *(WHO, n.d.)*

On the other hand, the number of donors born in Patagonia or Cuyo is very low compared to the high number born in the NOA or NEA. This is a reflection of the internal migratory flows in our country as reflected in the latest population census (Table 18).

		residence					
birth	region	centre	nea	noa	whose	patag	tot
	centre	22.167.769	146.898	167.688	156.979	295.676	22.935.010
	nea	1.050.158	3.388.659	32.821	10.366	57.174	4.539.178
	noa	850.936	24.318	4.174.139	62.855	64.874	5.177.122
	whose	267.193	4.487	49.515	2.848.567	89.588	3.259.350
	patag	204.369	6.199	9.582	24.263	1.707.417	1.951.830
	tot	24.540.425	3.570.561	4.433.745	3.103.030	2.214.729	37.862.490

Table 18: Migrations in Argentina by region Own elaboration based on data from Census 2010 **(INDEC, 2010)**

In the group of Patagonian donors, there were four cases of Chagas disease, one of which came from the province of Santa Cruz, a province with no risk of transmission by vinchuca (map 23). It would be necessary to investigate this person further to find out if between his departure from Patagonia and the date of donation he was not in an endemic area. But if this is not the case, we would be dealing with a case that is out of the ordinary for this disease.

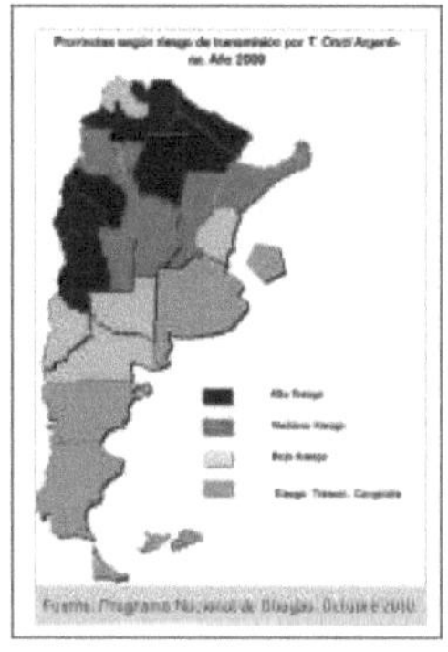

Map 23: Argentine provinces according to risk of T. cruzi transmission *(Dure & col, sf)*

(Dure & col, sf), since both the National Chagas Plan in 2010 and the WHO four years later declared this province to be free of the disease. At the time of donation, the donor was 37 years old and had also had hepatitis B.

In contrast, among donors from Cuyo and Patagonia, there were no cases of TLV, HIV or HCV. The case of HIV is surprising given that the HIV, AIDS and STI programme has higher rates in these regions than in the central region *(Direction de Sida, ETS, Hepatitis y TBC, Secr. de Gob. de Salud, Min.o de Salud y Desarrollo Social. Argentina, 2018).* In contrast, the results for HTLV were expected because the endemic areas are located in the north of the country (*Fujiyoshi & col, 2004; Gastaldello & col, 2004)*.

Returning to Chagas disease, Figure 24 shows that those born in CABA account for only 5.19% of positive cases. CABA is not an area of vector-borne transmission; there is only congënita transmission (map 23). Among these 37 cases, there could be children born to Chagasic mothers who were not detected at birth, or they could be people who travelled to an endemic area and became infected there. We do not have the data to be able to say which of the two categories they fall into.

The majority of Chagas positives are born in Northern Argentina or in neighbouring countries (approximately 76% of cases), coinciding with the endemic regions shown in map 21).Despite the fact that, as a country, we are in a low prevalence region for HBV (map 22), there is a considerable number of HBV infections born in the NOA, and Central Region (table 12 and graph 25) coinciding with what is shown in the 2014 MSAL report *(Angeleri & col, sf).* This report places Cuyo among the regions with the highest prevalence. However, in this work there are few cases from this region. Also, the total number of donors from that origin is low. But there is a large number of positive cases among those born in other countries of America, bordering (Paraguay and Bolivia) or not bordering (Peru), as mentioned above. Although there are very few cases, when added together they exceed the number of cases in the central region, so they should not be underestimated when designing prevention campaigns, especially since the vaccine has been included in the compulsory vaccination schedule *(RM 940/2000)*.

We know that the Americas region has the lowest global prevalence for the two hepatitis viruses of interest to us in the Blood Bank *(WHO , 2017)*, so any migratory flow from the "old world" can bring positive cases. In our experience this happened, for HBV, with European and East Asian donors (table 12). What was surprising was that we did not have any positive cases from

African migrants despite the recent influx of Senegalese migrants to CABA *(Cybel, 2018; Klipphan, 2019))*.

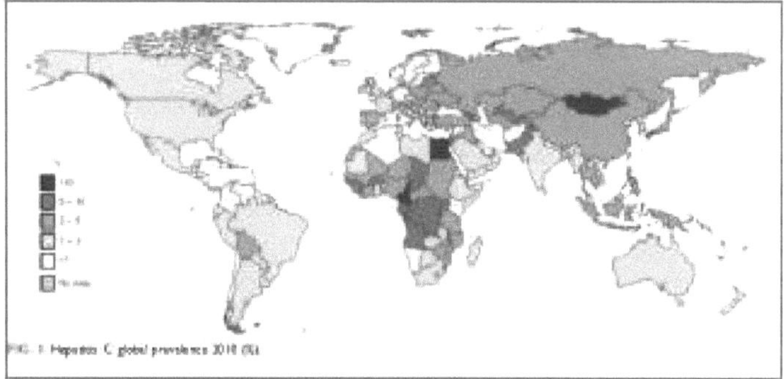

Map 24: HCV prevalence *(Lavanchy, 2011)*

This is because no member of this community has come to donate blood at our Bank or to collections from the Network that were referred to this service for processing. Nor have any cases of HCV been observed in donors born outside South America (table 12 and map 24), despite having received donors from places where the prevalence is higher than in Argentina *(Lavanchy, 2011)*.

To conclude this chapter, it can be observed that the cases of Brucellosis (graph 23) are concentrated in donors born in CABA and secondly, born in the province of Buenos Aires. Both together represent 62.79% of the positive cases for this infection. In this case, unlike the previous ones, internal migration does not seem to be a determining factor in its distribution.

Taking the variable "declared address" we can observe that slightly more than 94% of donors live in CABA or the first cordon of GBA (graph 29). Within the remaining small portion of donors, there are even a few foreigners who came to donate blood while they were in the city for tourism or work. In this group living outside Capital Federal and Conurbano there were no cases of Brucellosis, HCV, HIV or HTLV (graphs 31, 34, 35 and 36 respectively).

26.39% of Donors are domiciled in the programme area of the Hospital, if calculated over the total number of Donors domiciled in CABA (map 5, table 13). This value drops to 11.71% if calculated over the total number of donors. This could be interpreted in two ways. First, let us take into account that the population of communes 1, 2 and 14 together represent 21.39% of the city's population *(INDEC, 2010)*. The collections made by the Transfusion Medicine Network attract donors beyond the programme area to which the hospital belongs. This is because the "collection" device goes to workplaces (company offices, churches), places of study (universities, secondary schools) or simply places of transit (public squares, passenger transfer centres), in order to attract donors. But this alone is not enough to interpret these numbers, as the percentage of collection volunteers out of the total number of donors is still low *(Gendler & Trinca, 2015)*.

The other aspect to take into account is that the homes of hospitalised patients with transfusion requirements (and why not, their group of relations, meaning family members, friends and work colleagues), far exceed the hospital's programme area. These addresses cover not only the entire city of Buenos Aires, but also the Greater Buenos Aires (GBA), as shown in map 13. This is consistent with the official statistics of the GCBA *(General Directorate of Statistics and Censuses GCABA)* which reported for years that, in the hospitals of the GCABA, more than 40% of hospital admissions corresponded to patients coming from that province.

In summary, only 44.37% of donors are domiciled in CABA (Figure 29). As for the positive cases for the different TTIs (graphs 30 to 36), we see a similar distribution CABA/province. Expressed as a percentage of the total number of positives, we observe close but slightly lower values for S^filis (41.04%), Chagas (35.48%) and HCV (39.64%), slightly higher values for Brucellosis (49.61%) and higher values for HBV (52.06%), HIV (58.62%) and HTLV (71.42%). To try to understand this difference in distribution, we studied what happens in the interior of each of the subdivisions of the most representative large districts: the communes of CABA and the districts of GBA.

Only one third of the Donors domiciled in CABA (table 13) live in the programme area of the hospital. But positive cases for the different TTIs exceed this proportion, especially for S^filis, Chagas and HTLV, which represent 46.83, 41.5 and 36.66 percent respectively of the total number of positive cases domiciled in CABA for these TTIs (Figure 37). This concentration of cases becomes more evident if we only look at the portion of each bar in the graph that corresponds to commune 1 or look at maps 6 to 12. As we already know, in this commune there are precarious settlements, important in terms of number of inhabitants. These are villas 31 and 31 bis, which are home to numerous migrants from endëmic areas of S^filis, *(Arbo, 2010; Ortiz & col, 2018; Aguilar & col, 2018; Aguilar & col, 2016; San Miguel & col, 2010; Mini de Salud y Deportes, sf)* Chagas *(Meza, 2016), (Dir. G.ral de Vigilancia de la Salud, Paraguay, 2018), (Marquez Roa & col, 2013)*, HBV *(Centro Nac. de Epidemiologla, Prevention y Control de Enfermedades, 2016))* and HTLV *(Gotuzzo Herencia & col, 2010)*.

As mentioned above, no cases of HTLV were detected among donors living in Palermo (commune 14 and map 12). This does not mean that there are none, only that due to its low prevalence it is possible that they have not been detected because the members of the carrier group simply have not been sensitised by any donation campaign.

The highest number of positive cases of syphilis in CABA (map 6) is found in commune 1, followed by commune 14 and the southern communes of the city (3, 4 and 8). These last three are the least socio-economically developed *(INDEC 2010)*. Something similar happens in the GBA, where the highest number of positives is found in the district of La Matanza (map 14), which is also the most populous, and at the same time also has low rates of socio-economic development *(INDEC 2010)*. It is followed by Lomas de Zamora, Moreno, J. C. Paz, and others, within the conurbano, in terms of number of positives.

The number of cases of Brucellosis in commune 13 is striking, followed by communes 3 and

6, which are equal to commune 1, given that these are not areas related to livestock breeding, the dairy or meat processing industries. Paradoxically, commune 9, where the Mercado de Hacienda de Liniers is located *(Mercado de Liniers SA, sf)*, has only one case of Brucellosis. Among the Donors domiciled in the Province of Buenos Aires, something similar happens: the cases of Brucellosis are concentrated around the big cities (the suburbs of CABA and La Plata) but no cases were detected in the Donors of the interior of the province, despite the fact that cattle are raised there (Figure 40). The cases found could be related to the marketing of food that does not comply with all health regulations *(Scialfa & col, sf; Dibarboraa & col, 2017)*.

CABA is not an endemic area for Chagas disease. Despite this, there are numerous positive cases in communes 1 and 8 (see map 8). Cross-referencing the results obtained for domicile with those for birth, it can be seen that the aforementioned municipalities are those with the highest percentages of those born in areas of high Chagas prevalence (Bolivia and Paraguay (map 21) and provinces such as Salta, Jujuy, Santiago del Estero, Tucuman and Chaco (map 23), representing 40.92% and 38.84% of the donors domiciled in these municipalities.

The municipality of Palermo has a high number of Chagasic donors, but it also has a high number of eligible donors because it is the municipality of the hospital where this study is being carried out. This results in a lower concentration of cases compared to the common ones mentioned above. Similar causes would explain the high number of positive cases of Chagas disease among donors domiciled in the 24 districts of the GBA (see table 16).

With regard to HBV (map 9), the communes with the highest number of cases, in decreasing order, are 1, 3, 14, 4 and 5. If we relate this to the place of birth of donors in these districts (Table 14), we see that many of them (mainly those living in the retirement district) come from areas of high or medium endemicity such as the provinces of Salta and Jujuy *(Alonso S & col, 2019) and* from countries such as Peru *(Cabezas Sanchez, 2008)*, Paraguay *(Rovira & col, 2009)* and Bolivia *(Leon & col, 1999)*. In the GBA (table 16) we also see a significant number of donors born in the countries and provinces mentioned above, but the high number of donors from the districts of La Matanza and Lomas de Zamora suggests that the latter is the reason for the high number of hepatitis B donors in these districts.

As for the other hepatitis investigated, that caused by virus C, there is a notable concentration of cases in commune 15 (which includes the neighbourhoods of Chacarita, Villa Crespo, La Paternal, Villa Ortuzar, Agronom^a and Parque Chas) and secondly in commune 14. Due to the low number of cases (7 and 6 respectively), when cross-checking the data on address and place of birth, as was done with other markers, no clear pattern is seen with respect to the latter variable. What is striking is that all these cases belong to the male sex, (as opposed to cases reported in other communes, which also involve women) and most of them are over 40 years of age.

In terms of GBA (map 18), donors from Lomas de Zamora and La Matanza have the highest number of HCV positives. This is followed by 3 de Febrero and Malvinas Argentinas. La Matanza has the highest number of donors (3249) and 3 de Febrero the lowest (900) of these four districts (Table 16). This shows that the distribution of this infection does not have a uniform distribution in the conurbation of the city of Buenos Aires, so to know the true prevalence it would be necessary to carry out field tests in each district.

On the other hand, no positive cases were detected in donors from Ezeiza or San Isidro, despite being geographically contiguous to other districts where cases were detected. In these cases donor contributions were also low (400 and 571 respectively).

Finally, the commune with the highest number of HIV cases detected was commune 1, followed by communes 3, 4, 7 and 12 (map 11). With the exception of the latter, these are communes with low average incomes *(Bartfay N & col, 2017)*. In the GBA, slightly more than half of the cases domiciled in the province of Buenos Aires are concentrated in the southern area of the GBA (graph 39, table 15 and map 11), mostly in the district of Lanus.

Another interesting fact is obtained when crossing the addresses with the places of birth of the HIV-positive cases: a large proportion of them were born where they live. This is seen both for CABA (12 of the 36 cases were born in the city and 6 in GBA) and for the Province of Buenos Aires (52.17% of the cases were born and live in the Province of Buenos Aires). This means that the carriers of these viruses, with the exception of cases born in Paraguay, are mostly not migrants, which differentiates them from those infected by other TTIs such as Chagas.

HTLV cases are too few to make an analysis. The only thing that can be highlighted is the association for CABA with the presence of people born in Peru. This association is not seen in those domiciled in GBA.

To conclude the analysis of the data obtained, we will conclude with the analysis of co-infections. These occurred in 0.22% of donors, where the most frequent was HBV-Chagas, coinciding with the situation in Colombia (Cruz Bermudez & Moreno Collazos, 2015). However, unlike in that country, HBV-sii'ilis is in second place here. In third place was the infection by the two hepatitis viruses, followed by the syphilis-Chagas disease duo.

Associations with HIV were rare as shown in the literature *(Navarro, et al., 2008).* The most frequent was IBV (with 3 cases), while with HCV there was only one case.

Regarding HTLV, in contrast to the report by Cruz Bermudez *(2014)*, which mentions co-infection with s^filis in the first place, here the most frequent infection is with HBV, perhaps due to the high proportion of Peruvian-born donors among positive donors.

The largest number of cases included 2 infections although there were 3 cases of 3 positive markers, representing 3% of co-infections, implying that triple infections are extremely rare.

Concluding remarks

This paper has described which TTIs are most frequently detected as a result of the mandatory screening of blood donors assisted in this blood bank, their associations, and their variation over the years. Due to the requirements for blood donation they do not represent the actual prevalence in the general population but serve as an indirect measure to identify trend changes in their group membership.

Each group of infected persons has also been characterised according to their age group as well as their residence and place of birth. This will allow the formulation of hypotheses that will serve as a basis for future research of anaHtic character. It can also be used for the design of policies for the prevention of transmission and/or monitoring of those infected by the microorganisms studied.

Annexes

1. General workflow of the blood bank

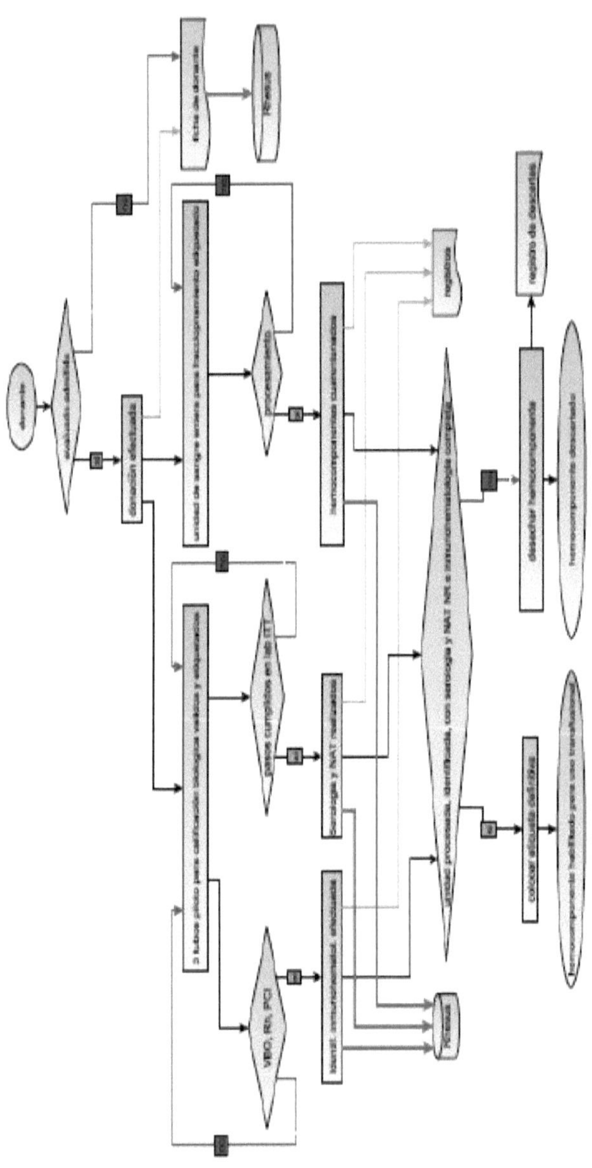

2. **Clinical Medical Interview Form of the Blood Banks of the GCABA Hospitals**

1. page 1 of the form

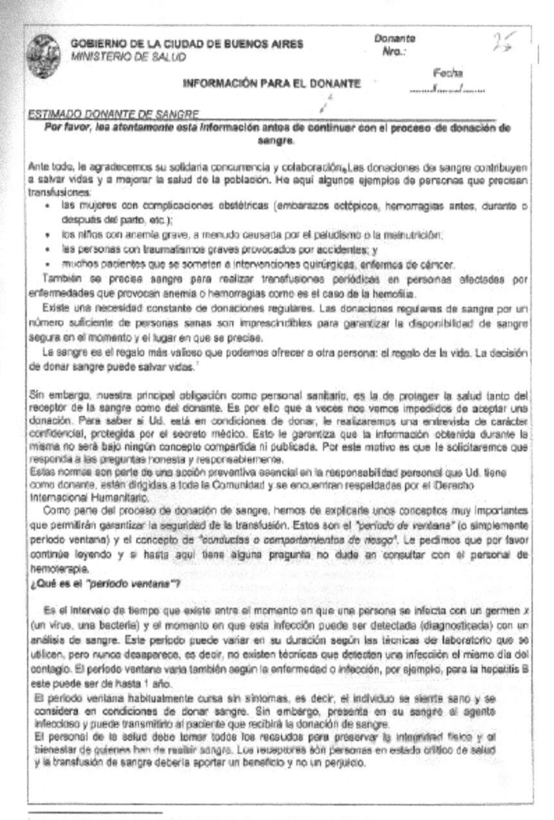

GOBIERNO DE LA CIUDAD DE BUENOS AIRES
MINISTERIO DE SALUD

Donante Nro.: 25

Fecha ..../......../........

INFORMACIÓN PARA EL DONANTE

ESTIMADO DONANTE DE SANGRE

Por favor, lea atentamente esta información antes de continuar con el proceso de donación de sangre.

Ante todo, le agradecemos su solidaria concurrencia y colaboración. Las donaciones de sangre contribuyen a salvar vidas y a mejorar la salud de la población. He aquí algunos ejemplos de personas que precisan transfusiones:

- las mujeres con complicaciones obstétricas (embarazos ectópicos, hemorragias antes, durante o después del parto, etc.);
- los niños con anemia grave, a menudo causada por el paludismo o la malnutrición;
- las personas con traumatismos graves provocados por accidentes; y
- muchos pacientes que se someten a intervenciones quirúrgicas, enfermos de cáncer.

También se precisa sangre para realizar transfusiones periódicas en personas afectadas por enfermedades que provocan anemia o hemorragias como es el caso de la hemofilia.

Existe una necesidad constante de donaciones regulares. Las donaciones regulares de sangre por un número suficiente de personas sanas son imprescindibles para garantizar la disponibilidad de sangre segura en el momento y el lugar en que se precise.

La sangre es el regalo más valioso que podemos ofrecer a otra persona: el regalo de la vida. La decisión de donar sangre puede salvar vidas.[1]

Sin embargo, nuestra principal obligación como personal sanitario, es la de proteger la salud tanto del receptor de la sangre como del donante. Es por ello que a veces nos vemos impedidos de aceptar una donación. Para saber si Ud. está en condiciones de donar, le realizaremos una entrevista de carácter confidencial, protegida por el secreto médico. Esto le garantiza que la información obtenida durante la misma no será bajo ningún concepto compartida ni publicada. Por este motivo es que le solicitaremos que responda a las preguntas honesta y responsablemente.

Estas normas son parte de una acción preventiva esencial en la responsabilidad personal que Ud. tiene como donante, están dirigidas a toda la Comunidad y se encuentran respaldadas por el Derecho Internacional Humanitario.

Como parte del proceso de donación de sangre, hemos de explicarle unos conceptos muy importantes que permitirán garantizar la seguridad de la transfusión. Estos son el *"período de ventana"* (o simplemente período ventana) y el concepto de *"conductas o comportamientos de riesgo"*. Le pedimos que por favor continúe leyendo y si hasta aquí tiene alguna pregunta no dude en consultar con el personal de hemoterapia.

¿Qué es el *"período ventana"*?

Es el intervalo de tiempo que existe entre el momento en que una persona se infecta con un germen *x* (un virus, una bacteria) y el momento en que esta infección puede ser detectada (diagnosticada) con un análisis de sangre. Este período puede variar en su duración según las técnicas de laboratorio que se utilicen, pero nunca desaparece, es decir, no existen técnicas que detecten una infección el mismo día del contagio. El período ventana varía también según la enfermedad o infección, por ejemplo, para la hepatitis B este puede ser de hasta 1 año.

El período ventana habitualmente cursa sin síntomas, es decir, el individuo se siente sano y se considera en condiciones de donar sangre. Sin embargo, presenta en su sangre el agente infeccioso y puede transmitirlo al paciente que recibirá la donación de sangre.

El personal de la salud debe tomar todos los recaudos para preservar la integridad física y el bienestar de quienes han de recibir sangre. Los receptores son personas en estado crítico de salud y la transfusión de sangre debería aportar un beneficio y no un perjuicio.

[1] Adaptado de Organización Mundial para la Salud - http://www.who.int/features/qa/61/es/

1

Preguntas habituales:

- *¿no se analizan a todas las bolsas (unidades) de sangre donadas?* Sí, todas las unidades de sangre son analizadas para detectar infecciones por VIH (o HIV), hepatitis B, hepatitis C, virus HTLV I- II, sífilis, Chagas y brucelosis. Pero si Ud. donó su sangre estando el "período de ventana" para alguna de ellas los análisis correspondientes arrojaran resultados NEGATIVOS, a pesar de usted tener la infección en cuestión. Estas unidades serán entonces consideradas aptas para ser transfundidas pero acabarán por contagiar al receptor.

¿Por qué los test de laboratorio no siempre consiguen detectar infecciones? TODAS las pruebas de laboratorio tienen un límite de sensibilidad por debajo del cual les es imposible detectar la infección. Aún los más sensibles tienen cierta limitación. Para poder confiar en un test de diagnóstico es necesario "haber dejado el período ventana atrás". Para ello se considera la fecha de la ultima exposición a una infección (si es que la hubo) y el tiempo de duración de su período ventana específico. Por ejemplo, tener sexo sin preservativos con una persona de la cual se desconoce si es portador de VIH representa una posible exposición. A partir de esa fecha de calculan 12 meses y a partir de entonces, un test de detección de VIH arrojaría un resultado confiable. (NOTA: el período ventana para VIH en mucho más corto, pero en la práctica se extiende a 12 meses para mayor seguridad de los receptores de sangre).

- *¿Si la sangre se conserva durante varias semanas... por qué no vuelven a analizarla antes de transfundirla?* Lo que permite la detección de la mayoría de las infecciones son unas moléculas llamadas *anticuerpos*. Estos se producen como respuesta a la presencia de un agente extraño dentro del cuerpo del huésped y para su producción son imprescindibles reacciones que solo pueden llevarse a cabo si la sangre esta aún en el cuerpo. En otras palabras, la sangre, una vez extraída del cuerpo del donante y puesta en una bolsa, queda como *"freezada"* y ya nada cambiará.

- *¿Cómo se puede reducir el "período ventana" para aumentar la seguridad transfusional?* La única forma es a través de una entrevista en profundidad realizada por profesionales del Banco de Sangre, quienes en forma individual y confidencial preguntarán sobre las situaciones de mayor riesgo para contraer infecciones graves que se transmiten por sangre y/o por vía sexual. El cuestionario se adecúa a la Legislación Nacional e Internacional vigentes y sigue las recomendaciones de la Organización Mundial de la Salud. Estas normas son parte de una acción preventiva con base en la responsabilidad que Ud. tiene como donante y están dirigidas a la comunidad en su conjunto. Se encuentran respaldadas por el Derecho Internacional Humanitario y son de carácter no discriminatorio.

¿Qué son las *"conductas o comportamientos de riesgo"*?

Las conductas o comportamientos de riesgo son practicas específicas que incrementan dramáticamente el riesgo de contraer una enfermedad o infección determinada. Así como fumar es una conducta de riesgo que multiplica de manera muy marcada las posibilidades de contraer cáncer de pulmón, la ingesta de sal en exceso es una conducta de riesgo coronario. Cuando consideramos la donación de sangre, nos interesa indagar en nuestros potenciales donantes sobre conductas o comportamientos de riesgo que aumenten las chances de adquirir una infección transmisible de donante a receptor durante una transfusión. Por ejemplo, en el caso del VIH, las conductas de riesgo pueden ser de índole sexual (sexo sin preservativos, parejas sexuales múltiples) o no-sexual (usar drogas inyectables y compartir jeringas).

En la actualidad la comunidad científica identifica conductas de riesgo distribuidas homogéneamente en la comunidad. Es por ello que este cuestionario no profundiza en cuestiones relacionadas con la identidad de género, la orientación sexual, el sexo transaccional, etc. Sí, en cambio, hace foco en conductas habituales y difundidas en la poblacion en su totalidad.

Las prácticas sexuales a cambio de dinero, drogas o alguna otra prestación son de riesgo para contraer infecciones como el VIH, Hepatitis B, Hepatitis C, sífilis, entre otras, si son coercivas, es decir, si una de las partes es sometida y privada del derecho a, por ejemplo, optar por el uso de preservativos. Las relaciones sexuales bajo la influencia de drogas y/o alcohol también son de alto riesgo por sí mismas. Las relaciones sexuales con múltiples parejas, aún con la utilización de preservativos, también representan un alto riesgo de infección.

Preguntas habituales:

- ¿Por qué aún con preservativos el sexo puede ser de riesgo? Si bien el preservativo es importante para protegernos durante las relaciones sexuales, no es 100% seguro. El personal del Banco de Sangre debe asegurarle al receptor que las unidades de sangre a ser transfundidas tienen la mayor seguridad posible. Las relaciones sexuales en situaciones de riesgo, aún con uso de preservativo, no garantizan la seguridad transfusional.

- ¿Que conductas serian de riesgo?

A continuación se detallan situaciones que son consideradas de alto riesgo para contraer infecciones graves transmisibles durante una transfusion de sangre y que deben ser consideradas con el solo objetivo de aumentar la seguridad transfusional.

- ✓ El uso de drogas prohibidas inyectables, consumo –inhalación- de cocaina
- ✓ El contacto a través de lesiones de piel o mucosas, con sangre y/o fluidos corporales de personas que desconocen su estado de salud en relacion a infecciones transmisibles por sangre,
- ✓ Las transfusiones frecuentes de componentes sanguineos.

En cuanto a las relaciones sexuales...:

- ✓ El sexo desprotegido (sin uso de preservativos), ya sea oral, vaginal o anal, fuera del contexto de una pareja estable y monogama, con o sin eyaculacion, con o sin uso de metodos anticonceptivos (recordar que estos previenen el embarazo pero no las enfermedades de transmision sexual).

Aun el sexo con preservativos puede ser de riesgo si...:

- ✓ Incluye cambio frecuente de parejas sexuales o es con parejas múltiples.
- ✓ Es con personas que cambian frecuentemente de parejas sexuales o tienen parejas múltiples, como ser el caso de los trabajadores sexuales o personas con adicciones que cambian sexo por drogas,
- ✓ Se trata de relaciones sexuales ocasionales.
- ✓ Es con personas portadoras de los virus de VIH, hepatitis o HTLV.
- ✓ Si es con personas en plan de hemodiálisis o que reciben transfusiones de componentes sanguineos.

Ultimas consideraciones a tener en cuenta

Algunas personas se deciden a donar sangre con la oculta intención de tener su sangre analizada para distintas enfermedades. Si es este su caso, le rogamos que por favor nos lo informe, podemos referirlo al laboratorio del hospital donde se le realizaran los análisis que usted desee sin poner en riesgo la salud de los receptores. Actualmente existen test rápidos que son gratuitos y entregan los resultados en unos pocos minutos. No tema, hable abiertamente de este tema con el técnico, el sabrá entenderlo.

Si luego de haber donado cree que puede estar en un "periodo ventana" para alguna infección, por ejemplo, al enterarse que su pareja sexual tiene una enfermedad, comuníquese lo antes posible con el personal del laboratorio donde dono su sangre. Muchas veces es posible "rescatar" su unidad de sangre donada y asi evitar el contagio durante una transfusión.

Si usted cree que su sangre podría no ser segura pero no puede ser abierto con respecto a ello porque, por ejemplo, sus familiares aguardan en la sala de espera a que usted done sangre, confíe en el personal de salud, nadie lo juzgara: simplemente marque con una X la *"ficha confidencial"* que se le entregó, en donde dice *"no debemos utilizar su sangre"*, y nosotros procederemos a descartarla de manera confidencial.

Una vez extraída, su sangre será analizada para hepatitis B y C, virus HTLV, Chagas, VIH, Brucelosis y Sífilis. Llegado el caso de que alguno de los análisis arrojara un resultado distinto al esperado, nos comunicaremos con usted por teléfono para invitarlo a volver e informarle sobre el hallazgo y ponerlo en contacto con profesionales de la salud para que continúen con la atención del problema que lo aqueja.

Hasta aquí usted ha leído todo lo que necesita saber en relación a la seguridad de la donaciones de sangre. Le agradecemos su atención. Si desea continuar con el proceso, de aviso al técnico de hemoterapia a cargo. El próximo paso incluye un cuestionario que usted deberá responder junto con el. Reiteramos más una vez el pedido de responder a las preguntar con absoluta sinceridad.
Muchas gracias.

DECLARACIÓN Y CONSENTIMIENTO LIBRE E INFORMADO DEL DONANTE

Hoy he concurrido a donar sangre u otro hemocomponente por mi libre y propia voluntad. Estoy en conocimiento que la donación de sangre es un acto solidario y altruista, por lo tanto, no he recibido ningún tipo de remuneración o incentivo Al hacerlo consiento que se me efectúan las pruebas necesarias para detectar infecciones transmisibles por sangre.
Voluntariamente autorizo que en caso de detección de cualquier hecho que esta institución considere relevante en relación a mi sangre se me notifique, al domicilio que he declarado. También entiendo que al existir el riesgo de transmitir enfermedades por mi sangre se registrará esta situación, y no debo donar en ningún establecimiento hasta tanto no exista una nueva autorización profesional especializada y que puedo ser transmisor de enfermedades aunque los análisis sean negativos.
He sido informado y he comprendido que durante o después de la donacion, eventualmente, puedo sufrir una reacción inesperada y fortuita, como por ejemplo, un hematoma alrededor del sitio de entrada de la aguja, la punción de una arteria, pérdida temporaria del conocimiento. He leído la información pre y post- donación que se me ha brindado; he tenido la oportunidad de consultar todo lo que he necesitado saber y me han respondido satisfactoriamente con términos comprensibles para mí. Dejo constancia que respondí a todas las preguntas con la verdad y con lo mejor de mi conocimiento. Es por ello que considero que estoy en condiciones de donar sangre u otro hemocomponente.

	<u>*Si el donante es menor de Edad*</u>
Firma del Donante-----------------------	*Firma del Tutor------------------* *Aclaración y N° DNI:-------------*

DATOS PERSONALES DEL DONANTE

Posta Colecta

Apellidos /Nombres ....

DNI / CI / LE / LC/Pasaporte N º..Nacionalidad..............................

Edad................ Fecha Nacimiento .... Lugar de Nacimiento.....................................

Domicilio Actual..Localidad...............................Código Postal............

Teléfono..Dirección de E-MAIL...

Donación Autóloga: ☐
Donación por Aféresis: ☐

NO RELACIONADO			DE REPOSICIÓN		
NUEVO	ULTERIOR		NUEVO	ULTERIOR	
	Habitual	No Habitual.		Habitual	No Habitual.

Lugar y fecha de la última donación: ....

¿Tuvo alguna reacción post donación? SI ☐ NO ☐

¿Fue diferido alguna vez como donante? SI ☐ NO ☐

Si es mujer, ¿Está embarazada o lo ha estado en las últimas 8 semanas? SI ☐ NO ☐

Cesárea ☐ parto Normal ☐ **¿Cuantos embarazos ha tenido?** ☐

La transfusión de plasma proveniente de mujeres multíparas se ha relacionado con una mayor probabilidad de presentar una injuria pulmonar aguda relacionada con la transfusión.

Firma del Donante..

GOBIERNO DE LA CIUDAD DE BUENOS AIRES *MINISTERIO DE SALUD* **HISTORIA CLINICA PRE-DONACIÓN**	*Donante Nro.*	
	Fecha ...../...../.....	

Información al donante	**SI**	**NO**
1-¿Considera que el Banco de Sangre le ha proporcionado información clara y entendible sobre la donación de sangre y las situaciones de riesgo para infecciones transmisibles durante una transfusión de sangre?		
2- ¿Ha leído atentamente todo el material y lo ha entendido?		
3- ¿Presenta alguna duda sobre lo que ha leído?		
En el día de hoy		
4- ¿Se siente bien? ¿Se siente "sano"?		
5- ¿Esta donando sangre de manera voluntaria?		
Antecedentes		
6- ¿Ha donado sangre en las últimas 8 semanas?		
7- Si la respuesta anterior es SI... ¿ha sufrido algún inconveniente posterior a la donación (desmayo, otros)?		
8- ¿Lo han rechazado como donante alguna vez, o le han dicho que *"Ud. no puede donar"*?		
9- Si la respuesta anterior es SI... ¿cuál fue el motivo?		
10- ¿Tomo aspirina o analgésicos en los últimos 3 días?		
11- ¿Ha tomado medicación para tratamiento de psoriasis, acné o enfermedades de la próstata?		
12- ¿Está tomando o ha tomado algún otro medicamento? ¿Cuál?		
13- ¿Ha padecido o padece enfermedades cardiovasculares (infarto, angina de pecho)?		
14- ¿Sufre de hipertensión arterial? ¿Qué medicación toma?		
15- ¿Sufre o ha sufrido de hemorragias o problemas de coagulación?		
16- ¿Ha padecido alguna enfermedad grave que haya exigido control médico periódico?		
17- Si la respuesta anterior es SI... qué enfermedad ha sido esta?		
18- ¿Ha sufrido de coloración amarillenta de piel o mucosas, cambios en el color de la orina y la materia fecal, junto con decaimiento general, fatiga, fiebre?		
19- ¿Ha dado "positivo" para un test de hepatitis?		
20- ¿Ha sufrido alguna enfermedad grave de pulmón (como asma), riñón, tiroides, aparato digestivo u otras?		
21- ¿Ha sufrido de episodios repetidos de desmayos, crisis de epilepsia y/o convulsiones?		
22- ¿Ha presentado episodios de fatiga, sudoración nocturna, fiebre prolongada, pérdida de peso sin motivo aparente, tos de larga duración?		
23- ¿Se ha hecho algún estudio para la tuberculosis?		
24- ¿Ha dado "positivo" o "*indeterminado*" en algún test para VIH (HIV)/SIDA en el pasado?		
25- ¿Tiene ganglios palpables, lesiones en la piel o mucosas que no hayan sido vistos aun por un médico?		
26- ¿Padece diabetes tratada con insulina?		
27- ¿Ha padecido cáncer? ¿Qué tipo?		
28- ¿Ha recibido quimioterapia y/o radioterapia?		
29- ¿Ha tenido algún problema hemorrágico o enfermedad de la sangre (anemia, leucemia)?		
30- ¿Le han diagnosticado enfermedad de Chagas o ha dado "positivo" en un test para Chagas?		
31- ¿Ha padecido paludismo/malaria en los últimos 3 años?		
32- ¿Ha visitado en el último año algún país donde el paludismo/malaria es endémico?		
33- ¿Ha recibido una transfusión de sangre o trasplante de tejido/órgano proveniente de otra persona?		
34- ¿Usted o algún familiar sufre o ha sufrido la enfermedad de Creutzfeldt- Jakob?		
35- ¿Ha recibido hormona de crecimiento de origen humano antes de 1987?		
36- ¿Ha recibido vacunacion o tratamiento para la rabia?		
37- ¿Ha recibido otras vacunas? ¿Cuáles? ¿Cuándo?		

38- ¿Ha usado drogas prohibidas inyectables, por ejemplo heroína?		
En las últimas 2 semanas:		
39- ¿Ha presentado fiebre, dolor de cabeza y malestar general?		
40- ¿Ha recibido tratamiento odontólogo? ¿Cuál?		
En el último mes		
41- ¿Ha estado en contacto con alguna persona que padeciera una enfermedad infectocontagiosa?		
En los últimos 6 meses		
42- ¿Ha concurrido a la consulta de algún médico o ha estado hospitalizado?		
43- Si la respuesta anterior es SI... ¿Cuál fue el motivo de consulta?		
44- ¿Ha sido sometido a algún tipo de endoscopia o cirugías no complicadas?		
En los últimos 12 meses		
45- ¿Ha sido intervenido quirúrgicamente y/o recibió sangre u otro componente?		
46- ¿Ha inhalado cocaína?		
47- ¿Se ha realizado tatuajes, perforación no estéril de piel (aros, piercing) y/o acupuntura		
48- ¿Ha estado en contacto con sangre o secreciones de otra persona por pinchazo accidental o salpicadura?		
49- ¿Mantuvo relaciones sexuales de riesgo para infecciones que se transmiten por sangre/sexo?		
50- ¿Ha estado en alguna(s) de las situaciones de riesgo para infecciones que se transmiten por sangre/sexo de las que se mencionan en la sección *"Información para el donante"*?		
51- Ha tenido sexo anal sin uso preservativo, ya sea como miembro insertivo (activo) o receptivo (pasivo) de la pareja?		
52- Ha tenido sexo vaginal sin uso de preservativo con una pareja no estable y monógama?		
53- ¿Convive o ha convivido, mantiene o ha mantenido contacto con alguien que padeciera hepatitis, tuberculosis o es portador de los virus de la hepatitis o el SIDA (VIH)?		
54- ¿Ha sido tratado para alguna enfermedad de transmisión sexual, como sífilis, gonorrea, clamidia, entre otras?		
55- ¿Ha sido víctima de violación, abuso sexual o cualquier forma de contacto sexual contra su voluntad?		
Si usted es mujer		
56- ¿Está embarazada?		
57- ¿Si esta o ha estado embarazada, cual es el número total de gestas?		
58- ¿Ha sufrido un aborto o tenido un parto en los últimos 12 meses?		
Estancias en el extranjero		
59- ¿Ha residido en un país extranjero? ¿Cuál? ¿Cuándo?		
60- Si la respuesta anterior es SI ¿Se ha relacionado sexualmente o ha incurrido en conductas sexuales de riesgo durante su estadía en dicho país?		
61- ¿Ha vivido durante más de un año (sumando todos los períodos de permanencia) en el Reino Unido (Inglaterra, Gales, Escocia, Irlanda del Norte, Islas del Canal, Isla de Man) entre 1980 y 1996?		
Por último		
62- ¿Confirma usted que la motivación para donar sangre no proviene de la necesidad de conocer su serología para VIH?		
63- ¿Confirma usted que no ha recibido dinero ni ningún otro tipo de compensación para donar sangre?		
64- ¿Confirma usted que ha entendido todas las preguntas que se le han formulado?		
OBSERVACIONES		

Firma del Donante...Documento Nº ....

ADMITIDO POR HISTORIA CLÍNICA: SI ☐ NO ☐ Causa médica definitiva Cód.........

Causa médica temporaria Cód..................

Observaciones:...

....

Firma y Sello del Personal que Realizó la Entrevista

CONTROL CLINICOS

Hto / Hb................TA:.......................Pulso:...............Temp.:...............Peso:...............

Inspección de los brazos:..

Observaciones:

ADMITIDO EN Control CLÍNICOS: SI ☐ NO ☐

Operador:..

EXTRACCION

Tipo de Bolsa..............**N° de lote**..............**Anticoagulante** CFD | CFD-SAG-M Otro:......

N° de la tubuladura utilizada..

Fecha de vencimiento de la Bolsa.......................... **Brazo punzado:** D | I

Dificultad en la Extracción: SI | NO (Códigos: **SD** - **RV** - **Ag** - **T**- **Bo** - **Lp**)

Tolerancia al Procedimiento: Buena Regular Mala **Tipo de Reacción:** (Códigos: **He** - 1 – 2-)

Peso de la Bolsa:..............**Hora de iniciada la extracción**:..............**Hora de finalizada**...............

Muestras SI | NO

Operador..

OBSERVACIONES...............................

....

FIRMA DEL RESPONSABLE DEL PROCESO HEMODONACIÓN

NOTA: **SD** (se retira sin donar) -**RV** (red venosa)- **Ag** (aguja)- **T** (tubuladura)- **Bo** (bolsa)- **Lp** (lipocimia).
He (hematoma)- 1 (leve-moderada)- 2 (sever

General workflow of the Donor Sector of the Blood Bank

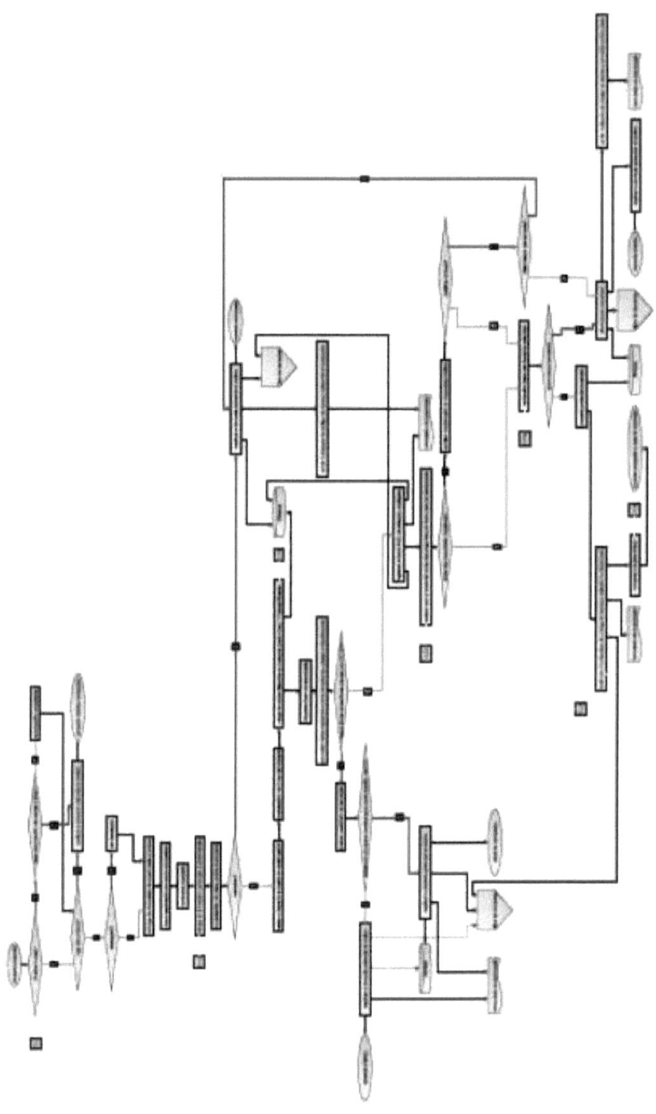

3. Project Approval

CABA, 14 de Abril de 2018

Considero que el proyecto de Tesis "Prevalencia de Infecciones de Transmision Transfusional estudiadas en donantes del Banco de Sangre Intrahospitalario del Hospital Juan A. Fernández, del Gobierno de la Ciudad Autónoma de Buenos Aires en el periodo 2006-2017 y su relevancia en la gestion del Servicio de Hemoterapia" esta en condiciones de ser presentado para su segunda evaluación

Mg. Silvina Bering
Docente Adscripta
Dto. de Salud Pública
Facultad de Medicina
UBA

CABA, 14 April 20 i 8

I consider that the Thesis project "Prevalence of Transfusion Transmitted Infections studied in donors of the Intra-Hospital Blood Bank of the Juan A. Fernandez Hospital, of the Government of the Autonomous City of Buenos Aires in the period 2006-2017 and its relevance in the management of the Henniotherapy Service" is ready to be submitted for its second evaluation.

Mg. Siivtna Bering
Doeenie Attaché Oto. de Salud Publica racultad de Medinina
VBA

5. Approval of the ERC

GOBIERNO DE LA CIUDAD DE BUENOS AIRES
HOSPITAL GENERAL DE AGUDOS JUAN A. FERNÁNDEZ
COMITÉ DE ÉTICA EN INVESTIGACIÓN

Buenos Aires, 30 de mayo 2019

Ref. Protocolo: PREVALENCIA DE INFECCIONES DE TRANSMISIÓN TRANSFUSIONAL ESTUDIADAS EN DONANTES DEL BANCO DE SANGRE INTRAHOSPITALARIA DEL HGAJAF DEL GCBA EN EL PERÍODO 2006-2017 Y SU RELEVANCIA EN LA GESTIÓN DEL SERVICIO DE HEMOTERAPIA

Nº CODEI: 201822
Investigador principal: Dra Gendler

Estimado/a Investigador/a:

Por la presente le informamos que el Comité de Ética en Investigación del Hospital Fernandez ha otorgado la renovación anual a vuestro protocolo de referencia.

Le recordamos que, según los Procedimientos Operativos de este Comité; *"Los investigadores serán responsables de remitir la información sobre el avance del estudio bajo su responsabilidad y sobre cualquier contingencia que ocurra ajena a lo establecido por protocolo mediante alguno de los siguientes documentos: informe de avance o informe final". "El IP debe informar al CEIHF los avances producidos durante su investigación, anualmente"*

El CEIHF, en cumplimiento de sus funciones, realiza monitoreos del desarrollo de las funciones aprobadas.

LA PRESENTE NOTA DEBE SER IMPRESA Y ARCHIVADA EN LA CARPETA DEL INVESTIGADOR

PRESIDENTE COMITÉ DE ... INVESTIGACIÓN HOSPITAL FERN...

Atte, Dra Analia Cortes

Comite de Etica en Investigación Hospital Fernández (CEIHF)
Cerviño 3356 – 7º Piso. 1425 CABA
fernandez_cei@buenosaires.gob.ar
TE: 4808-2618

Página 1 de 1

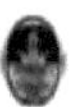

GOBIERNO DE LA CIUDAD DE BUENOS AIRES
HOSPITAL GENERAL DE AGUDOS JUAN A. FERNÁNDEZ
COMITÉ DE ÉTICA EN INVESTIGACIÓN

Buenos Aires, 4 de junio de 2018

Ref. Protocolo:
"PREVALENCIA DE INFECCIONES DE TRANSMISIÓN TRANSFUSIONAL ESTUDIADAS EN DONANTES DEL BANCO DE SANGRE INTRAHOSPITALARIA DEL HOSPITAL GRAL. DE AGUDOS J. A. FERNÁNDEZ DEL GCBA EN EL PERÍODO 2006-2017 Y SU RELEVANCIA EN LA GESTIÓN DEL SERVICIO DE HEMOTERAPIA".

N° CEIHF: 201822

Investigadoras: Bq. Silvina Gendler

Estimada Bq. Gendler

Por la presente les informamos que el Comité de Ética en Investigación del Hospital Fernández ha aprobado desde el punto de vista metodológico y ético la siguiente documentación perteneciente al protocolo de referencia.

1. Protocolo de investigación.

La aprobación tuvo lugar en la sesión ordinaria del día 4 de junio de 2018, Acta N° 786 con la presencia de la Dra. Graciela Bidvinik, Dra. María Laura Garau, Lic. Guillermo Cardozo, Sra. Mirta Castro, Sr. Gonzalo Vigo, Dra. Patricia Gitelman y Dra. Verina Edul.

La presente aprobación tiene una validez por un año, supeditada al cumplimiento de las obligaciones enumeradas a continuación:

1. Informar el inicio del estudio
2. Informar los desvíos al protocolo.
3. Presentar el informe final del estudio

El CEIHF, en cumplimiento de sus funciones, realiza monitoreos del desarrollo de las investigaciones aprobadas.

Si el estudio se extiende más allá del 4 de junio de 2019 se debe solicitar una extensión de la aprobación.

El estudio no puede comenzar hasta contar con la Disposición Autorizante de la Dirección del Hospital.

Atte.

Dra.
María
Laura
Garau

Comité de Ética en Investigación Hospital Fernández (CEIHF)
Cerviño 3356 – 7° Piso. 1425 CABA
fernandez_cei@buenosaires.gob.ar
TE. 4808-2618

6. Method of processing the database.

1. Rhesus
2. DONOR BOOK: Save as rtf x year
3. Copy/paste to Excel: special pasting: Unicode text
4. adding logical functions
5. add filters
6. add transposition
7. split screen vertically and horizontally
8. Colouring
a. From outside orange background
b. Deferred and ineligible: red letter
c. Self-Excluded Background on board
9. Copy rows to values
10. Pull out first columns
11. Extract in another window
a. From outside
i. HOSPITAL
ii. INSTITUTE
iii. FOUNDATION
iv. HEMOCENTRE
v. CEMIC
vi. MARIA FERRER
vii. MATERNITY
viii. ACADEMY
ix. OTHER
b. Deferred and ineligible:
c. Self-excluded
12. Order
a. Retrieved
b. From outside
c. Deferred
d. Self-excluded
13. Check match sum
14. Check for shortages
15. Unify all the years in 1 file for each type.
a. Extra^dos + self-excluded
b. From outside
c. deferred
16. deferred:
a. sort by type and year
b. masc/fem:
c. ages
d. add
i. delete unnecessary data
ii. spaces to match n° columns
iii. n/a (no data)

17. from outside:
a. sort by Htal of origin and year
b. spaces to match n° columns
c. n/a (no data)
18. extracted:
a. male/female
b. ages
c. unify
i. births
ii. homes:

1. communes/neighbourhoods CABA (https://www.buenosaires.gob.ar/comunas)

2. parties/cities other than CABA
d. delete unnecessary data
e. spaces to match n° columns
f. n/a (no data)
i.
g. take out
i. repeated
ii. incomplete
19. Setting up frames:
a. From outside
b. Deferred
c. extra^dos
20. Unify the databases of extra^dos and RR Excel file.
21. Disease/infection: classify according to outcome:
a. S^filis
i. Screening
ii. algorithm
iii. confirmation
b. Brucellosis
i. Screening
ii. algorithm
iii. confirmation
c. Chagas
i. Screening
ii. algorithm
iii. confirmation
d. Hepatitis b
i. Screening
ii. algorithm
iii. complementary/confirmatory
e. Hepatitis c
i. Screening
ii. algorithm
iii. complementary
f. HIV
i. Screening
ii. algorithm

iii. confirmation

g. HTLV

i. Screening

ii. algorithm

iii. confirmation

22. Unify the 3 components of the databases (external, extracted and deferred).
23. Complete with SD= no data
24. Numbering and titling
25. Add filters

6. Fine database

See attached CD

Bibliography

Aach, E., Szmuness, W., Mosley, J., Hollinger, F., Kahn, R., Stevens, C., ... Werch, J. (1981). Serum Alanine Aminotransferase of Donors in Relation to the Risk of Non-A,Non-B Hepatitis in Recipients The Transfusion-Transmitted Viruses Study. *N Engl J M 304*, 989-994.

Abbas Zaheer, H., Saeed, U., Waheed, Y., Karimi, S., & Waheed, U. (2014). Prevalence and Trends of Hepatitis B, Hepatitis C and Human Immunodeficiency Viruses among Blood Donors in Islamabad, Pakistan 2005-2013. *J Blood Disorders Transf, 5*(6), ISSN: 21559864 DOI: 10.4172/2155-9864.1000217.

Aguilar A, Estigarribia G, Gimenez L , Samudio T , Kawabata A, Lopez G, Jara M., Rolon R, Alvarenga F, Schwartz Benzaken A, Espinosa A, Munoz S. (2016). *Prevalencia de VIH y Sffilis y Conocimientos, Practicas y Attitudes de la Poblacion Indi'gena segun Familias Linguisticas en el Paraguay.* Retrieved from Ministerio de Salud Publica y Bienestar Social: http://onusidalac.org/1/images/informe-Estudio-indigenas-paraguay2016.pdf

Aguilar G, Kawabata A, Rolon R, Sosa D, Delgado K. (2018). *HIV Epidemiological Situation Report.* Retrieved from https://www.mspbs.gov.py/dependencias/pronasida/adjunto/62ddce-INFEPIVIH2018120720192.pdf

Alonso S, Aquino R, Coronel E, Ezcurra M, Levite V, Roitman K. (2019). *Boleti'n on viral hepatitis in Argentina N°1.* Retrieved on 25/12/19, from http://www.msal.gob.ar/images/stories/bes/graficos/0000001592cnt-2019- 10_boletin-hepatitis.pdf

Alter M, Kuhnert WL, Finelli L. (2003). *Guidelines for Laboratory Testing and Result Reporting of Antibody to Hepatitis C Virus.* Retrieved from https://www.cdc.gov/mmwr/preview/mmwrhtml/rr5203a1.htm

Alter, MJ; Margolis, HS; Bell, BP; Bice, SD; Buffington, J; Chamberland, M; . Coleman, PJ; Cummings, BA; Dentinger, CM; Garfein, RS; Hodgson, W; Braatz Ivie, K; Kelly Rima Khabbaz, MG; Lyerla, R; Mahoney, LD; Mast, EE; Moyer, LA; Sabin, KM; Shapiro. (16 October 1998). Recommendations for Prevention and Control of Hepatitis C Virus (HCV) Infection and HCV-Related Chronic Disease. *MMWR Recommendations and Reports, 47*(RR 19), 1-39nic. Retrieved 01/01/202020, from https://www.cdc.gov/mmwr/preview/mmwrhtml/00055154.htm

Amegeiras, B., Gonzalez, J., Jotimliansky, L., Zingoni, C., & Vulcano, C. (2013). *Viral load survey in geographic areas of Argentina with high prevalence of hepatitis B virus.* Retrieved on 12/22/2019, from http://www.actagastro.org/numeros- anteriores/2013/Vol-43-N1/Vol43N1-PDF09.pdf.

Angeleri P, Coronel E, Solari I, Vidiella G, Vulcano S, Bruno M; Giovacchini C, Buyaylsqui MP, Antman J, Varela T, Herrmann J. (2016). *Viral hepatitis Guia para los equipos de salud.* Retrieved on December 21, 2019, from http://www.msal.gob.ar/images/stories/bes/graficos/0000000780cnt-2016-09_hepatitis-virales-equipos-de-salud.pdf

Angeleri P, Levite V, Vidiella G. (n.d.). *Prevalence of viral hepatitis and syphilis in people undergoing prenuptial screening in Argentina.* (P. d. Ministry of Health, Ed.) Retrieved on 12/23/2019, from http://publicaciones.ops.org.ar/publicaciones/prev_control_enfermedades/Prenupcial HepatitsSifilis.pdf

Angeleri P, Pando MA, Solari J, Vidiella G. (n.d.). *Viral Hepatitis in Argentina.* (P. d. Ministry of Health, Ed.) Retrieved on 12/22/2019, from http://www.msal.gob.ar/images/stories/ryc/graficos/0000000865cnt-2014- 09_estado-hepatitis-virales-argentina.pdf

Angheben, A., Boix, L., Buonfrate, D., Gobbi, F., Bisoffi, Z., Pupella, S., ... Aprili, G. (2015). Chagas disease and transfusion medicine: a perspective from non-endemic countries. *Blood Transfus, 13*, 540-50 DOI 10.2450/2015.0040-15.

Antman J, Baldiviezo L, Bertolini, L, Buyayisqui MP, Codebo O, Couto P, Echenique A, Giovacchini G,

Stefanic N, Tapia J, Varela T. (2015). *Boleti'n Integrado de Vigilancia N° 244 SE 4 2015.* Retrieved on 12/23/2019, from https://www.argentina.gob.ar/sites/default/files/boletin-integrado-de-vigilancia-n244-se4.pdf.

Antman J, Giovacchini C, Baldiviezo L, Buyayisqui MP, Carrizo J, Codebo O, Couto P, Echenique A, Manana A, Mariscal E, Stefanic N, Tapia J, Varela T. (2016). *Boleti'n Integrado de Vigilancia N° 296 SE 5 2016.* Retrieved on 12/23/2019, from https://www.argentina.gob.ar/sites/default/files/boletin-integrado-de-vigilancia- n296-se5.pdf.

Arbeitskreis Blut, Untergruppe "Bewertung Blutassoziierter Krankheitserreger". (2010). *Human Cytomegalovirus (HCMV).* Retrieved on 23 December 2016, from https://doi.org/10.1159/000322141

Arbo, A. (2010). S^filis: alarming situation in Paraguay. *Rev. Inst. Med. Trop., 5*(1), 5-6. Retrieved on 12/23/2019, from http://scielo.iics.una.py/pdf/imt/v5n1/v5n1a01.pdf

Arrizabalaga, J. (2000). Las "enfermedades emergentes" en las postrimerias del siglo XX: El sida. *Politica y Sociedad*, 93-100. Retrieved from Dpto. de Historia de la Ciencia (IMF- CSIC). Barcelona. Polrtica y Sociedad, 35, Madrid (pp. 93-100) retrieved 14/12/19: https://core.ac.uk/download/pdf/38819182.pdf

Barin, F. (2000). Viruses and unconventional transmissible agents: update on transmission via blood Transfus. *Transfus. Clin. Biol., Jun; 7* (Suppl 1), 5s-10s. Retrieved from DOI: 10.1016/s1246-7820(00)80009-9

Barril, G., & Traver, J. (2003). Decrease in the hepatitis C virus (HCV) prevalence in hemodialysis patients in Spain: effect of time, initiating HCV prevalence studies and adoption of isolation measures. *Antiviral Res., 60*(2), 129-34. Retrieved from DOI: 10.1016/j.antiviral.2003.08.008

Bartfay N, Chaui J, El Ahmed Y, Fernandez M, De Florio F, Giboin Mazzola MA, Gonzalez Lebrero C, Janeiro E, Rodriguez M, Valenzuela M, Zyssholt M. (2017). *Analisis de Situation de Salud de la Ciudad Autonoma de Buenos Aires.* (M. d. Salud, Ed.) Retrieved on 12/22/2016, from https://www.buenosaires.gob.ar/sites/gcaba/files/asis_caba_2016_dic17_vf_1.pdf

Berini, C., Pascuccio, M., Bautista, C., Gendler, S., Eirin, M., Rodriguez, C., ... Biglione, M. (2008). Comparison of four commercial screening assays for the diagnosis of human T- cell Lymphotropic virus types 1 and 2. *Journal of Virological Methods, 147*, 322-327. Retrieved on 12/21/2019, from https://doi.org/10.1016/j.jviromet.2007.09.012

Biglione, M., & Berin, i. C. (2013). Aportes y consideraciones sobre la infeccion por los virus Linfotropico-T humanos tipo 1 y 2 en Argentina. *Buenos Aires, 21*(81), 84-94. Retrieved on 12/22/2019, from https://ri.conicet.gov.ar/bitstream/handle/11336/21367/CONICET_Digital_Nro.25649 _A.pdf?sequence=2&isAllowed=y

Boletm Oficial de la Ciudad Autonoma de Buenos Aires N° 2292. (01 September 2005). Law 1777/05. *Organic law of communes.* CABA. Retrieved 12/29, 2019, from https://www.buenosaires.gob.ar/areas/leg_tecnica/sin/normapop09.php?id=77544& qu

Boletm Oficial de la Republica Argentina, N° 147203 (18 September 2015). Resolution 1508/15 Ministry of Health of the Nation - National Blood Plan. *Prohibese la exigencia de donantes de sangre de reposicion.* Retrieved 01 01 01 2020, from https://www.boletinoficial.gob.ar/detalleAviso/primera/132942/20150918?busqueda =1

Boletm Oficial de la Republica Argentina, N° 24576 Page: 6. (31 Dec 1980). Law 22360/80. *Enfermedad de Chagas Interes National.* Retrieved on 12/29/2019, from https://www.boletinoficial.gob.ar/detalleAviso/primera/7082899/19801231?busqued a=1

Boletm Oficial de la Republica Argentina, N° 25313 (1983). Law 22990/83. *Ley National de Sangre.* Retrieved 27, 12. 2019, from https://www.boletinoficial.gob.ar/detalleAviso/primera/7090606/19831202?busqued a=1

Boletm Oficial de la Republica Argentina, No. 26972 (20 Sep 1990). Law 23798/90. *Public Health (AIDS)*. CABA. Retrieved on 12/29, 2019, from https://www.boletinoficial.gob.ar/detalleAviso/primera/7118835/19900920?busqued a=1

Boletm Oficial de la Republica Argentina, N° 29513 (27 October 2000). Resolution 940/00 Ministry of Health of the Nation. *Incorporase con caracter obligatorio al Calendario Nacional de Vacunacion la vacuna antihepatitis B*. Retrieved 01 01 2020, from https://www.boletinoficial.gob.ar/detalleAviso/primera/7209360/20001027?busqued a=1

Boletm Oficial de la Republica Argentina, N° 30497. (1 Oct 2004). Regulation of Law 22.990. *Decree 1338/04. Derogacion del decr. 375/89*. Retrieved 23 Dec. 12, 2019, from https://www.boletinoficial.gob.ar/detalleAviso/primera/7267148/20041001?busqued a=1

Boletm Oficial de la Republica Argentina, N° 31232 (5 Sept 2007). Law 26281/07. *Law for the prevention and control of all forms of transmission of Chagas Disease, until its definitive eradication from the entire national territory*. Retrieved on 12/29/2019, from https://www.boletinoficial.gob.ar/detalleAviso/primera/9179320/20070905?busqued a=1

Boletm Oficial de la Republica Argentina, No. 51282 (11 July 2013). Resolucion 797/13 Ministerio de Salud de la Nacion - Plan Nacional de Sangre. *Normas Administrates y Tecnicas y los Criterios de Selección de Donantes de Sangre.* Retrieved on 01 01 2020, from https://www.boletinoficial.gob.ar/detalleAviso/primera/90503/20130711?busqueda= 1

Boletm Oficial de la Republica Argentina, N° 9129. (19 February 2014). Resolution 139/14 Ministry of Health of the Nation - National Blood Plan. *Modifi'quese el segundo parrafo del punto P. bajo el titulo PREPARACION DE PRODUCTOS SANGUINEOS subti'tulo P.ITTdel Anexo I de la Resolution Ministerial 797/2013*. Retrieved 01 January 2020, from https://www.boletinoficial.gob.ar/detalleAviso/primera/102192/20140219?busqueda =1

Boletm Oficial de la Republica Argentina, N°147201 (18 September 2015). Resolution 1507/15 Ministry of Health of the Nation - National Blood Plan. *Modifi'quese el ANEXO I de la Resolution Ministerial N° 797/2013, Normas Administrates y Tecnicas*.
Retrieved on 01 01 01 2020, from https://www.boletinoficial.gob.ar/detalleAviso/primera/132941/20150918?busqueda =1

Boletm Oficial de la Republica Argentina, N°147213 (18 September 2015). Resolution 1509/2015, National Ministry of Health - National Blood Plan. *Apruebese el material de Information para el donante, documento para la autoexclusion pre- donacion, cuestionario personal del donante y autoexclusion confidential post- donacion*. Retrieved 01 01 01 2020, from https://www.boletinoficial.gob.ar/detalleAviso/primera/132943/20150918?busqueda =1

Official Gazette of the Government of the Autonomous City of Buenos Aires (2010). Decreto N° 087/10. *reglamentacion de la ley de Sangre de CABA* . Retrieved December 25, 2019, from https://documentosboletinoficial.buenosaires.gob.ar/publico/20100127.pdf

Official Gazette of the Government of the Autonomous City of Buenos Aires (2010). Law 3328/10. *Ley de Sangre de CABA*. Retrieved on December 25, 2019, from https://documentosboletinoficial.buenosaires.gob.ar/publico/20100127.pdf

Borgareto, M., Buceta, A., Stazzoni, C., & Torres, O. (2015). Main causes of Blood Donor deferral in the last 30 months. *Rev. Arg. de Transf, XLI* (3), 193. Retrieved on 12/25/2019, from https://www.aahitc.org.ar/wp- content/uploads/2015/11/RAT032015.pdf

Bouzas MB, Fay F, Canero Velasco MC, Coronel E, Solari J, Vidiella G, Angeleri P, Falistocco C. (n.d.). *Algorithms for the diagnosis of viral hepatitis Programa Nacional de Hepatitis Virales, Ministerio de Salud de la Nacion.* Retrieved on 12/27/2019, from http://www.msal.gob.ar/images/stories/bes/graficos/0000000684cnt-2015- 03_algorithms-hepatitis-2015.pdf.

Bouzas, M., Garay, M., & Arrigo, D. (November 2013). Session: Virology and diagnosis. (AAEEH, Ed.) *Consenso Argentino de Hepatitis C, book of abstracts*, pp. 63-66.

Buenos Aires City, Jefatura de Gabinete, Atencion y Gestion Ciudadana, Gestion Comunal, Comunas (n.d.). *Buscador de comunas*. Retrieved on 01/09/202020, from https://www.buenosaires.gob.ar/comunas

Busch, M. (2004). Should HBV DNA NAT replace HBsAg and/or anti-HBc screening of blood donors? . *Transfusion Clinique et Biologique, 11*, 26-32 doi:10.1016/j.tracli.2003.12.003. Retrieved on 12/22/2019, from http://www.em- consulte.com/en/article/22366

Cabezas Sanchez, C. (2008). Situation and control of hepatitis B and Delta in Peru. *Acta Med Per, 25*(2). Retrieved on 12/22/2019, from http://www.scielo.org.pe/pdf/amp/v25n2/a10v25n2.pdf

CDC/PAHO. (2011). *Chikungunya virus preparedness and response in the Americas ISBN: 978-92-75-31632-0.* (W. D. PAHO, Ed.).

Centers for Disease Control and Prevention (1999). Summary of notifiable diseases, United States, 1998. *MMWR* , *47*(53). Retrieved on 12/25/2019, from https://www.cdc.gov/mmwr/preview/index98.html

Centro Nacional de Epidemiolog^a, Prevencion y Control de Enfermedades (2016). *Boleti'n epidemiologico del Peru Epidemiological week N° 52 December 25 to 31 ISSN electronic version: 2415-0762.* Retrieved on 12/19/2019, from https://www.dge.gob.pe/portal/docs/vigilancia/boletines/2016/52.pdf

Cetiner, S., Duranb, A., Kibarb, F., & Yaman, A. (2017). Performance comparison of new generation HCV core antigen test versus HCV RNA test in management of hepatitis C virus infection Transfusion and Apheresis. *Science, 56*, 362-366. Retrieved on 12/22/2019, from https://www.sciencedirect.com/science/article/pii/S1473050217300290?via%3Dihub

Coluccl, M., Berini, C., Canepa, C., Ruggieri, M., Halperin, N., Rojas, F., ... Biglione, M. (2016). Chronic adult T-cell leukaemia: parenteral transmission of human T lymphotropic T virus type 1 at birth? *Hematologi'a, 20*(3), 344 - 348. Retrieved on 12/25/2019, from http://www.sah.org.ar/revista/numeros/14%20vol%2020%20N3- 2016.pdf.

Cooper, S., Schim van der Loeff, M., & Taylor, G. (2009). The neurology of HTLV-1 infection. *Practical Neurology, 9*, 16-26. Retrieved on 12/25/2019, from http://dx.doi.org/10.1136/jnnp.2008.167155

Coppola, N. (2001). Nuove frontiere diagnostiche in corso di Brucellosi. *Le Infezioni in Medicina, 3*, 130-136. Retrieved on 12/25/2019, from http://www.infezmed.it/media/journal/Vol_9_3_2001_1.pdf

Cruz Bermudez, H., & Moreno Collazos, J. (2015). Seroprevalence of Chagas screening and factors associated with coinfection in a Colombian blood bank during 2006-2011. *Rev. Med. Risaralda, 21* (1), 26-30. Retrieved on 12/28/2019, from https://revistas.utp.edu.co/index.php/revistamedica/article/view/9302/6591

Cruz Bermudez, H., Moreno Collazos, J., Restrepo Sierra, M., & Angarita Fonseca, A. (2014). Seroprevalence of screening for T-cell lymphotropic virus (HTLV) and factors associated with coinfection in volunteer blood donors in Colombia. *Salud Uninorte. Barranquilla (Col.), 30*(2), 95-103. Retrieved on 12/25/2019, from https://www.redalyc.org/pdf/817/81732428002.pdf

Cruz, JR. (2012). Working Standards for Blood Services Third Edition. Washington, D.C. (PAHO/WHO, Ed.) ISBN: 978-92-75-31643-6. Retrieved on 12/31/2019, from https://www.paho.org/hq/dmdocuments/2012/HSS-BloodServiceStandards2012.pdf

Cura EN, de Titto EH, Segura EL (1992). Quality control of immunodiagnosis of Chagas disease, Manual of procedures. In I. N. Chaben, *part 1.3 Serological methods* (pp. 9-13). Ministry of Health and Social Action of the Republic of Argentina and PAHO, Transmissible Diseases Programme.

Cybel, Y. (2018). *Senegalese in Buenos Aires From Senegal to Argentina. The cry from the south.* Retrieved on December 25, 2019, from http://elgritodelsur.com.ar/2018/06/senegaleses- manteros-represion.html

Programme Area Department (n.d.). *Ministry of Health, GCABA.* Retrieved 11 01 01 2020, from https://www.buenosaires.gob.ar/hospitalargerich/departamento-de- area-programatica

Department of Health Systems and Services. (2016). *Preliminary recommendations for blood services in the face of the Zika virus epidemic: its potential impact on the spread of infection and the availability and safety of blood and blood components. WHO/PAHO,Washington, D.C.* (PAHO, Ed.) Retrieved on 12/31/2019, from https://www.paho.org/hq/dmdocuments/2016/ZIKV-sangre-feb-16.pdf

Dibarboraa, M., Cappuccioa, J., Aznard, M., Bessonee, F., Piscitelli, H., & Pereda, A. y. (2017). Serological detection of Brucella suis, influenza virus and Aujeszky's disease virus in family pig farms of less than 100 dams in Argentina. *Rev. Argent Microbiol., 49*(2), 158---165. Retrieved on 12/28/2019, from https://doi.org/10.1016/j.ram.2016.09.010

Direccion de Estad^stica e Informacion de Salud, Ministerio de Salud y Desarrollo Social (n.d.). *Basic Indicators, Argentina.* Retrieved on 12/29, 2019, from http://www.deis.msal.gov.ar/index.php/indicadores-basicos/

Direccion de Sangre y Hemoderivados (s.f.). *Sacretaria de Gobierno, Ministerio de Salud y Desarrollo Social, Argentina.* Retrieved 11 01 01 2020, from http://www.salud.gob.ar/disahe/index.php?option=com_content&view=article&id=31 0&Itemid=59

Direccion de Sida, ETS, Hepatitis y TBC, Secretaria de Gobierno de Salud, Ministerio de Salud y Desarrollo Social. Argentina (2018). *Boleti'n on HIV, AIDS and STIs in Argentina .* Retrieved on 12/25/2019, from http://www.msal.gob.ar/images/stories/bes/graficos/0000001385cnt-2018-12-20_boletin-epidemiologico-vih-sida-its_n35.pdf.

Direccion General de Estad^stica y Censos GCABA. (n.d.). *Hospital discharges of the Government of the City of Buenos Aires and percentage distribution by habitual residence. City of Buenos Aires. Anos 1994/2018 .* Retrieved on 12/25/2019, from https://www.estadisticaciudad.gob.ar/eyc/?p=28906

Direccion General de Estad^stica y Censos, GCBA. (2010). *Households and population censused in private dwellings and households and population with Unsatisfied Basic Needs (UBN) by commune. City of Buenos Aires.* Retrieved 12/29/2019, from INDEC. Censo Nacional de Poblacion, Hogares y Viviendas 2010 : https://www.estadisticaciudad.gob.ar/eyc/?p=24187

Direccion General de Estad^stica y Censos, Gobierno de la Ciudad de Buenos Aires (2016). *Areas programticas de salud. City of Buenos Aires.* Retrieved on 01/13/2020, from https://www.estadisticaciudad.gob.ar/eyc/?p=57915

Direccion General de Vigilancia de la Salud, Ministerio de Salud Publica y Bienestar Social Paraguay (2018). *Boletin Epidemiologico SE 1 A LA SE 4 Nro. 4.* Retrieved on 12/14/2019, from http://vigisalud.gov.py/files/boletines/SE4_2018_Boletin.pdf

Direccion Provincial de Estad^stica, Ministerio de Econom^a, Pcia. As. (n.d.). *El metodo de las Necesidades Basicas Insatisfechas (NBI).* Retrieved on 12/29, 2019, from http://www.estadistica.ec.gba.gov.ar/dpe/index.php/sociedad/condiciones-de- vida/necesidades-basicas-insatisfechas/177-metodologia-necesidades-basicas- insatisfechas/230-metodologia-necesidades-basicas-insatisfechas.

Voluntary Blood Donation (n.d.). *Red de Medicina Transfusional, Programas y Redes de Salud, Ministerio de Salud, GCABA.* Retrieved 11 January 2020, from https://www.buenosaires.gob.ar/salud/programasdesalud/donacion-voluntaria-de- sangre/red-de-medicina-transfusional.

Dure I, Cuba C, Hidalgo SE. (n.d.). *Course on vector-borne diseases for community agents in environment and health. Module V: Chagas disease. Ministry of Health Argentina.* Retrieved on 12/28/2019, from http://www.msal.gob.ar/images/stories/bes/graficos/0000000172cnt-08-2-3-3-I-modulo-Chagas.pdf

Echenique A, Giovacchini C, Mariscal E, Carrizo Olalla J, Medici JM, Tapia J, Baldiviezo L, Buyayisqui MP, Ferro N, Stefanic N, Varela T. (2017). *Boletin Integrado de Vigilancia I N° 345- SE 04 Secretaria de Promotion y programas sanitarios MSAL Argentina ISSN 2422-698X.* Retrieved on 12/28/2019, from https://www.argentina.gob.ar/sites/default/files/boletin_integrado_de_vigilancia_n34 5-se4.pdf

El cronista (n.d.). *GBA map.* Retrieved on December 28, 2019, from https://www.cronista.com/__export/1505785948607/sites/diarioelcronista/img/2017 /09/18/distritos_crop1505785948404.jpg_258117318.jpg

Establishments - Hospitals and Health Centres. (n.d.). *Ministry of Health, GCABA*. Retrieved 11 Jan. 01, 2020, from https://www.buenosaires.gob.ar/salud/establecimientos

Faddy, H. M., Fryk, J. J., Watterson, D., Young, P. R., Modhiran, N., Muller, D. A., ... Marks, D. C. (2016). Riboflavin and ultraviolet light: impact on dengue virus infectivity. *Vox Sanguinis, 111,* 235-241 DOI: 10.1111/vox.12414.

Fainboim H, Marciano S, Di Benedetto N, Gadano A. (2013). Argentine consensus on hepatitis B AAEEH. *Acta Gastroenterol Latinoam, 43*, 59-74. Retrieved on December 25, 2019, from https://www.redalyc.org/pdf/1993/199326065013.pdf

Fakile, Y., Jost, H., Hoover, K., Gustafson, K., Novak-Weekley, S., Schapiro, J., ... Park, I. (2018). Correlation of treponemal immunoassay signal strength values with reactivity of confirmatory treponemal testing. *J Clin Microbiol 56:e 2018 01165- 17 DOI: 10.1128/JCM.01165-17.*

Fay, O., Gonzalez, J., & Rey, J. (2005). Haemodonants and the general population. *Acta Gastroenterol Latinoam;, 35*(Suppl N°1), 11-12. Retrieved on 12/25/2019, from http://www.redalyc.org/articulo.oa?id=199323385002

Fujiyoshi, T., Li, H.-C., Lou, H., Yashiki, S., Karino, S., Zaninovic, V., . . . and Tajima, K. (2004). Characteristic Distribution of HTLV Type I and HTLV Type II Carriers among Native Ethnic Groups in South America. *AIDS Research and Human Retroviruses, 15*(14). Retrieved on 12/25/2019, from https://doi.org/10.1089/088922299310124

Garda, M. D., Mulazzi, R., Quiroga, V., Lorenzini, A., Rey, J. A., & Vellicce, A. F. (2018). Donor deferral in a blood bank in the city of Buenos Aires. *Rev. Arg de Transf Vol. XLIV / N° 3-4, XLIV*(3-4), 235 / 242. Retrieved on 12/25/2019, from https://www.aahitc.org.ar/wp-content/uploads/2018/11/Revista-Argentina-de- Transfusi%C3%B3n-3-4-2018.pdf.

Gastaldello, R., Hall, W., & Gallego, S. (1 March 2004). Seroepidemiology of HTLV-I/II in Argentina: an overview. *J Acquir Immune Defic Syndr., 35*(3), 301-8. Retrieved on 12/25/2019, from https://insights.ovid.com/crossref?an=00126334-200403010-00012

GCABA. (n.d.). *Buenos Aires City*. Retrieved 11 January 2020, from https://www.estadisticaciudad.gob.ar/eyc/

GCBA, D. G. (2010). *Households and population censused in private dwellings and households and population with Unsatisfied Basic Needs (UBN) by commune. City of Buenos Aires.* Retrieved on 12/29/2019, from Direccion Gsobre la base de datos de INDEC. Censo Nacional de Poblacion, Hogares y Viviendas 2010: https://www.estadisticaciudad.gob.ar/eyc/?p=24187

Gendler, S. (2005). Anti-HCV Antibody Screening: Results from 12 Years of Experience. Part One: i. Are improvements in reagent quality sufficient? *Revista Argentina de Transfusion vol XXXI N*4*, 181-186.

Gendler, S. (2013). Prevalence of Brucellosis in Blood Donors in a public hospital in CABA. *Rev. Arg. de Infectol. Dr. F. J. Muniz, 16* (suppl1), 29.

Gendler, S. A., & Trinca, A. (2015). Evaluation of the sensitivity and specificity of reagents for the determination of antibodies for Chagas disease in Blood Banks. *Rev. of Bioq. and Pathol. Clin., 79*(No. 2 May-Aug.), 30-38. Retrieved on 12/25/2019, from http://www.aba-online.org.ar/ejemplares-revista-bypc-2015/revista-n-79-2-mayo- August.

Gendler, S., & Estevez, D. (2017). Cost-benefit evaluation of CMV screening in a BSI of a CABA public hospital. *Rev. Arg. de Transf., XLIII*(3), 191-192. Retrieved on 12/25/2019, from https://www.aahitc.org.ar/wp- content/uploads/2017/10/Revista-Argentina-de-Transfusi%C3%B3n-3-2017-.pdf.

Gendler, S., & Pascuccio, M. (2007). Routine HIV screening among blood donors in Buenos Aires (Argentina): results from six years' experience and report of a single windowperiod donation. *Rev. de Enf. Infec. y Mbiol. Clin 25(2):82-90; DOI: 10.1157/1309856.*

Gendler, S., & Trinca, A. (2013). Influence of voluntary donation on discards by serolog^a: evolution in a public hospital of the GCABA. *Rev. Arg. de Transf, XXXiX* (3), 122. Retrieved on 12/25/2019, from https://www.aahitc.org.ar/rat/RAT032013.pdf

Gendler, S., Milano, V., Camino, S., del Turco, V., Zanetti, V., Alvarez, A., ... Lena, N. (2011). Seroreactivities in blood banks of public hospitals in the city of Buenos Aires. *Revista argentina de transfusion,, 37*(3), 196. Retrieved on 12-25-2019, from https://www.aahitc.org.ar/rat/RAT032011.pdf

Gendler, S., Trinca, A., Estevez, D., & Baston, M. (2014). HBV; HCV and HIV in blood banking: impact of the epidemiological profile of the blood donor and the introduction of nucleic acid technology on the safety of blood components. *Rev. Sci. HGAJAF, 17* (2), 2-7.

Government of the Autonomous City of Buenos Aires (n.d.). *Buenos Aires, city*. Retrieved on 01/11/2020, from https://www.buenosaires.gob.ar/

Gomes, R., Ferreira do Nascimento, E., & Carvalho de Araujo, F. (2007). Por que os homens buscam menos os servigos de saude do que as mulheres? As explicates de homens com baixa escolaridade e homens com ensino superior. *Cad. Saude Publica, Rio de Janeiro, 23*(3), 565-574. Retrieved on December 25, 2019, from http://www.scielo.br/scielo.php?script=sci_abstract&pid=S0102-311X2007000300015&lng=en&nrm=iso&tlng=pt

Gonzalez, E., Birnenbaum, S., Suarez, A., & Caggiano, S. (2017). Analysis of the causes of deferral in voluntary blood donors. *Rev. Arg. de Transf Vol. XLIII / N° 3, XLIII* (3), 208. Retrieved on 12/25/2019, from https://www.aahitc.org.ar/novedades/revista-argentina-de-transfusion-n3-ano-2017/

Gonzalez, J., Rey, J., & Marozzi, F. (November 2013). Session: Epidemiology and prophylaxis. Conference: Prevalence in the general population and in blood donors. (AAEEH, Ed.) *Argentine Consensus on Hepatitis C. Book of abstracts*, pages 38-42.

Gonzalez, JE; Fainboim, H, Frider, B; Ramonet, M; Tanno, H; Canero Velasco, MC; Rey, J; Terg, R; Lestrem, MD; A, Chiera; Munoz, A; Daruich, J; Ciocca, M; Trigo, P. (2016). *Epidemiologia Informe N°16 Servicio Hepatitis y Gastroenteritis, Departamento Virologia, Laboratorio Nacional e Referencia, Instituto Nacional de Enfermedades Infecciosas (INEI), Administration National de Laboratorios e Institutos de Salud (ANLIS), "Dr.* . Retrieved on 12/25/2019, from http://www.hepatitisviral.com.ar/wp-content/uploads/2017/10/informe-16.pdf

Gonzalez, V., Fernandez, G., Dopico, E., Margall, N., Esperalba, J., Munoz, C., ... Matas, L. (2015). Evaluation of the Vitros Syphilis TPA chemiluminescence immunoassay as a first-line method for reverse syphilis screening. *J Clin Microbiol*, 53:1361-1364. doi:10.1128/JCM.00078-15.

Gotuzzo Herencia, E., Gonzalez Lagos, E., Verdonck Bosteels, K., Mayer Arispe, E., Ita Nagy, F., & Clark Leza, D. (2010). Twenty years of research on HTLV-1 and its medical complications in Peru: Overview. *Acta Med Per, 27*(3), 196203. Retrieved on 12/28/2019, from https://www.researchgate.net/publication/262756599_Veinte_anos_de_investigacion _on_HTLV-1_and_its_medical_complications_in_Peru_Peru_General_Overviews.

Gregoire, Y., Germain, M., & Delage, G. (May 4, 2018). Factors associated with a second deferral among donors eligible for re-entry after a false-positive screening test for syphilis, HCV, HBV and HIV. *Vox sang , Vol113,* , 339-344. Retrieved on December 29, 2019, from https://onlinelibrary.wiley.com/doi/10.1111/vox.12644

Hofstraat, S. H., Falla, A. M., Duffel, I. E., Amato-Gauci, A. J., Veldhuijzen, I. K., & Tavoschi, L. (2017). Current prevalence of chronic hepatitis B and C virus infection in the general population, blood donors and pregnant women in the EU/EEA: a systematic review. *Epidemiol. Infect., 145*, 2873-2885 doi:10.1017/S0950268817001947. Retrieved on 12/29/2019, from https://www.ncbi.nlm.nih.gov/pmc/articles/PMC5647665/pdf/S0950268817001947a. pdf.

INDEC, Republica Argentina (n.d.). *National Institute of Statistics and Census*. Retrieved 11 Jan 2020, from https://www.indec.gob.ar/indec/web/Institucional-Indec- BasesDeDatos-6

National Institute of Statistics and Census (2010). *National Census of Population, Households and Dwellings*. Retrieved on 12/29, 2019, from https://www.indec.gob.ar/indec/web/Nivel4-Tema-2-41-135

Irfan, S., Uddin, J., Abbas Zaheer, H., Sultan, S., & Baig, A. (2013). Trends in Transfusion Transmitted Infections Among Replacement Blood Donors in Karachi, Pakistan Turk. *J Hematol , 30*, 163-167 DOI: 10.4274/Tjh.2012.0132. Retrieved on 12/29, 2019, from https://www.ncbi.nlm.nih.gov/pmc/articles/PMC3878468/pdf/TJH-30-163.pdf

Kamb, M; Schwartz Benzaken, A; Karem, K; Matheu, J; Perez (2015). *Guidance for syphilis diagnosis in latin america and the caribbean: how to improve adoption, interpretation and quality of diagnosis in different clinical settings.* Department of Communicable Diseases and Health Analysis, PAHO/WHO, Washington, DC. Retrieved on 12/30/2019, from http://iris.paho.org/xmlui/bitstream/handle/123456789/7707/9789275318607_esp.pdf?sequence=1&isAllowed=y

Karimi, G., Zadsar, M., & Akbar Pourfathollah, A. (2017). Seroprevalence and geographical distribution of human T-Lymphotropic virus type 1 among volunteer blood donors in endemic areas of Iran. *Virology Journal*, 14:14 DOI 10.1186/s12985-017-0693-9. Retrieved on 12/29/2019, from https://virologyj.biomedcentral.com/articles/10.1186/s12985-017-0693-9

Khan, H., Hill, A., Main, J., Brown, A., & Cooke, G. (2017). Can Hepatitis C Virus Antigen Testing Replace Ribonucleic Acid Polymearse Chain Reaction Analysis for Detecting Hepatitis C Virus? *Open Forum Infect Dis., Spring; 4(2): ofw252. doi: 10.1093/ofid/ofw252*. Retrieved on 12/29/2019, from https://www.ncbi.nlm.nih.gov/pmc/articles/PMC5445222/pdf/ofw252.pdf

Kim, A., Lee, Y., Kim, K., Chu, Y., Baik, b., Kim, E., ... Pi, S. (2006). Transfusion-related Cytomegalovirus Infection Among Very Low Birth Weight Infants in an Endemic Area. *J Korean Med Sci, 21*, 5-10 ISSN 1011-8934. Retrieved on December 29, 2019, from https://synapse.koreamed.org/Synapse/Data/PDFData/0063JKMS/jkms-21-5.pdf

Klipphan, A. (2019). *Human trafficking in Argentina: the route of Senegalese eyeglass-sellers-turned-slaves.* Retrieved on 12/29, 2019, from https://www.infobae.com/sociedad/policiales/2019/03/31/trafico-humano-en- argentina-la-ruta-de-los-senegaleses-vendedores-de-anteojos-convertidos-en- esclavos/

Kozel, A; Martmez, LE; Taraborrell, i D; Carvalho, N. (2017). El sistema agroalimentario del Area Metropolitana de Buenos Aires al 2030/2050. (INTA, Ed.) *coleccion investigacion, desarrollo e innovacion, 1° ed,* pag 11 ISBN 978-987-521-869-7. Retrieved 12/29/29/219, from https://www.academia.edu/37183586/El_sistema_agroalimentario_del_%C3%81rea_Metropolitana_de_Buenos_Aires._Exploratorio_exercicio_exploratorio_de_prospectiva_territorial.

Laplagne, A., Picon, M., Mohammad, S., Moreno, M., Varga, B., Pacheco, S., & Garramuno, M. (2015). Valoracion del impacto de la promocion en las postas de donantes IPHEM 2007 al 2015. *Rev. Arg. de*

Transf., XLI(3), 196. Retrieved on 12 29, 2019, from https://www.aahitc.org.ar/wp-content/uploads/2015/11/RAT032015.pdf

Lavanchy, D. (Feb 2011). Evolving epidemiology of hepatitis C virus. *Clinical Microbiology and Infection, 17*(2). Retrieved 17 Jan 2020, from https://www.clinicalmicrobiologyandinfection.com/article/S1198-743X(14)61648- 7/pdf

Legislature of the Province of Buenos Aires (1 June 2006). LAW N° 13.473. *Delimitation of the Conurbano Bonaerense*. Retrieved 12/29, 2019, from https://normas.gba.gob.ar/documentos/VrAGAiGB.pdf

Leon, P., Venegas, E., Bengoechea, L., Rojas, E., Lopez, J., Elola, C., & Echevarria, J. (1999). Prevalence of hepatitis B, C, D and E virus infections in Bolivia. *Rev. Panam Salud Publica/Pan Am J Public Health, 5*(3). Retrieved on 12/29/2019, from https://www.scielosp.org/pdf/rpsp/1999.v5n3/144-151/es

Lia, J., Caoa, Y., Hinmanb, S., McKeatingc, K., Guana, Y., Hua, X., & Cheng, Q. Y. (February 15, 2018). Efficient label-free chemiluminescent immunosensor based on dual functional cupric oxide nanorods as peroxidase mimics. *Biosensors and Bioelectronics, Volume 100*, 304-311. Retrieved on December 29, 2019, from https://www.sciencedirect.com/science/article/pii/S0956566317306188?via%3Dihub

Liumbruno, G., & Franchin, M. (January 2015). Solvent/detergent plasma: pharmaceutical characteristics and clinical experience. *Journal of Thrombosis and Thrombolysis, 39*(1), 118-12. Retrieved on December 29, 2019, from https://link.springer.com/article/10.1007%2Fs11239-014-1086-1#citeas

Lucero, NE, (1994). *Techniques for the diagnosis of Brucellosis.* Inst. Nac. de microbiolog^a Carlos G Malbran.

Lucero, NE; Escobar, GI; Ayala, SM; Hasan, DB (2008). Manual of Procedures: Techniques for the Diagnosis of Human Brucellosis. Brucellosis Service, National Institute of Infectious Diseases, A.N.L.I.S. "Dr. Carlos G. Malbran" - WHO Global Salm Surv Regional Reference Centre for South America. Retrieved 09 01/09/202020, from file:///D:/Users/Silvina/Scritorio/BIBLIOG%20TESIS/bibliog/ManualProcedimientos Brucelosis_2008.pdf

Lya, T., Lapercheb, S., Brennanc, C., Vallaric, A., Ebela, A., Huntc, J., ... Devarec, S. (15 December 2004). Evaluation of the sensitivity and specificity of six HIV combined p24 antigen and antibody assays. *Journal of Virological Methods, 122*, 185-194 doi:10.1016/j.jviromet.2004.08.018. Retrieved on December 29, 2019, from https://www.sciencedirect.com/science/article/abs/pii/S0166093404002599?via%3Di hub

Marquez Roa, N., Lemir de Zelada, M., & Molas, A. (December 2013). Serologic frequency of Trypanosoma cruzi infection in donors. *Mem. Inst. Investig. Sci. Health, 9*(2), 26 31. Retrieved on 12/29, 2019, from https://revistascientificas.una.py/index.php/RIIC/article/view/96/40

Martin, M., Carrizo, L., Moyano, R., & Verde, E. (2017). External blood drives as a strategy to obtain voluntary donors. Our experience between 2012 and 2016. *Rev. Arg. de Transf, XLIII*(3), 203-204. Retrieved on 12/29/2019, from http://www.aahi.org.ar/wp-content/uploads/2017/10/Revista-Argentina-de- Transfusi%C3%B3n-3-2017-.pdf.

Mazeron, M. (June 2000). Leukodepletion and infection by cytomegalovirus. *Transfusion Clinique et Biologique, 7* (Supplement 1), 31s-35s. Retrieved from https://doi.org/10.1016/S1246-7820(00)80013-0

Mendez-Lozano, M., Rodriguez-Reyes, E., & Sanchez-Zamorano, L. (November-December 2015). Brucellosis, a zoonosis present in the population: a time series study in Mexico. *Saludpublica de Mexico, 57*(6), 519-527. Retrieved on December 29, 2019, from http://www.scielo.org.mx/pdf/spm/v57n6/v57n6a10.pdf

Mercado de Liniers SA (n.d.). Retrieved 18 Jan. 01, 2020, from

http://www.mercadodeliniers.com.ar/indexnuevo.htm
Meza, G. (2016). Seroprevalence of Chagas disease in pregnant women in the department of Cordillera before and after the implementation of prenatal Chagas control in the periods 1997 and 2011. *Mem. Inst. Investig. Sci. Health, 14*(3), 73-80 Doi: 10.18004/Mem.iics/1812-9528/2016.014(03)73-080.
Argentine Ministry of Health (n.d.). *Boleti'n epidemiologico.* Retrieved on December 23, 2019, from https://www.argentina.gob.ar/salud/epidemiologia/boletines2017
National Ministry of Health (August 2012). *Gulas para la atención al paciente infectado con Trypanosoma cruzi (Enfermedad de Chagas) 2° edicion Resolucion Ministerial 1337/14.* Retrieved on December 29, 2019, from http://www.msal.gob.ar/images/stories/bes/graficos/0000000622cnt-03-guia-para-la- atencion-al-paciente-con-chagas.pd
Ministry of Health and Sports. La Paz, Bolivia (n.d.). *Anuario estadistico en salud2009 23rd ed. ISBN : 978-99954-50-25-0.* Retrieved on 12/22/2019, from http://saludpublica.bvsp.org.bo/cc/BOX.79/documentos/nest15.pdf
Ministry of Health, Argentina (n.d.). *Direccion de Estadisticas e informacion en salud.* Retrieved 14 Jan. 01, 2020, from http://www.deis.msal.gov.ar/index.php/indicadores-basicos/
Monge-Maillo, B., Jimenez, C., Perez-Molina, J., Norman, F., Navarro, M., Perez-Ayala, A., ... Lopez-Velez, R. (Nov 2009). Imported Infectious Diseases in Mobile Populations, Spain. *Emerging Infectious Diseases - www.cdc.gov/eid - Vol. 15, No. 11, Nov 2009 DOI: 10.3201/eid1511.090718, 15*(11), DOI: 10.3201/eid1511.090718. Retrieved on 12/29/2019, from https://wwwnc.cdc.gov/eid/article/15/11/pdfs/09-0718.pdf
Moore, B. (April 1953). Complications of blood transfusion. *Caad. M. A. J, 68*, 332-337. Retrieved on December 29, 2019, from https://www.ncbi.nlm.nih.gov/pmc/articles/PMC1822765/pdf/canmedaj00679- 0015.pdf
Moral, M; Laplume, H; Sardi, F; Jacob, NR; Garro, S; Lucero, N; Reynes, E; Lopez, G; Samartino, L; Amiotti, P; Hart, J, Bagnat, E; Arejula, C; Antman, J; Giovachini, C; Casas, N. (November 2013). *Infectious diseases: brucellosis. Direccion de Epidemiologia, Ministerio de Salud de la Nacion ISSN 1852-1819.* Retrieved on December 30, 2019, from http://www.msal.gob.ar/images/stories/bes/graficos/0000000304cnt- guia-medica-brucelosis.pdf
Morales, J. (15 Nov 1996). Clinical aspects of Chagas disease. *Bol. Acad. Nac. de Medic. Supplement in homage to Dr. Salvador Maza*, 69-87 ISBN 0374-647x.
Morgan Freiman, J., Tran, T., Schumacher, S., White, L., Ongarello, S., Cohn, J., ... Denkinger, C. (Sep 06, 2016). HCV Core Antigen Testing for Diagnosis of HCV Infection: A systematic review and meta-analysis. *Ann Intern Med., 165*(5), 345-355. doi:10.7326/M16-0065. Retrieved on 12/30/2019, from https://www.ncbi.nlm.nih.gov/pmc/articles/PMC5345254/pdf/nihms852426.pdf
Mori, A., Ojima-Kato, T., Fuchi, S., Kaiya, S., Kojima, T., & Nakano, H. (2017). Development of a rapid immunoassay system: Luminescent detection of antigen-associated antibody-luciferase in the presence of a dye that absorbs light from free antibody-luciferase. *Journal of Bioscience and Bioengineering , 124*(6), 694-699. Retrieved on 12/30/2019, from http://dx.doi.org/10.1016/j.jbiosc.2017.06.016
Musso, D., Richard, V., Broult, J., & Cao-Lormeau, V. (Nov 2014). Inactivation of dengue virus in plasma with amotosalen and ultraviolet A illumination. *Transfusion, 54*(11), 2924-2930 DOI: 10.1111/trf.12713. Retrieved on 12/30/2019, from http://onlinelibrary.wiley.com/doi/10.1111/trf.12713/abstract
Nascimento, M., Mayaud, P., Cerdeira, S. E., Torres, K., & Francesch, S. J. (2008). Prevalence of Hepatitis B and C Serological Markers Among First-Time Blood Donors in Brazil: A Multi-Center Serosurvey. *journal of Medical Virology, 80*, 53-57. Retrieved on 12/30/2019, from

https://onlinelibrary.wiley.com/doi/epdf/10.1002/jmv.21046
Navarro, D., Panchuck, P., Villalba Salinas, V., Salazar, M., Merino, D., & Balbachan, S. (2008). Hepatitis B, C and HIV co-infection in a Blood Bank in Corrientes,
Argentina. *Rev. Cubana Med Trop, 60*(2), 181-3. Retrieved on 12/30/2019, from http://scielo.sld.cu/pdf/mtr/v60n2/mtr12208.pdf
Oliveira Cavalcanti Soares, C., Almeida Teles, J. A., dos Santos, A. F., Silva, S. O., Rocha Andrade Cruz, M., & da Silva-Junior, F. (Sept.-Oct. 2015). Prevalence of Brucella spp in humans. *Rev. Latino-Am. Enfermagem, 23*(5), 919-26 DOI: 10.1590/01041169.0350.2632. Retrieved on 12/30/2019, from http://www.scielo.br/pdf/rlae/v23n5/es_0104-1169-rlae-23-05-00919.pdf
WHO. (8 December 2015). Draft Global Health Sector Strategy on Sexually Transmitted Infections for 2016-2021. *Draft*. Retrieved on 12/31/2019, from https://www.who.int/reproductivehealth/GHSS_STI_SP_06012016.pdf
WHO/PAHO. (1 October 2014). *Resolution CD53.R6 plan of action for universal access to safe blood 66th session of the WHO regional committee for the americas Washington, D.C., USA, 29 September to 3 October 2014.* Retrieved on 12 31, 2019, from https://www.paho.org/hq/dmdocuments/2014/CD53-R6-s.pdf
PAHO. (2017). *Blood supply for transfusion in Latin American and Caribbean countries 2014 and 2015 Washington, D.C.; ISBN: 978-92-75-31958-1.* Retrieved on 12/31/2019, from http://iris.paho.org/xmlui/bitstream/handle/123456789/34082/9789275319581-spa.pdf?sequence=1&isAllowed=y
PAHO/WHO. (1999). Strengthening blood banks in the Region of the Americas. Resolution CD41. *41st Directing Council, 51st session of the Regional Committee*. San Juan, Puerto Rico. Retrieved 12/30/2019, from http://iris.paho.org/xmlui/bitstream/handle/123456789/1409/CD41.R15sp.pdf?seque nce=2
PAHO/WHO. (1 Aug 2005). Progress report on the regional blood safety initiative and plan of action for 2006-2010 CD46/16 (Eng.) Washington, D.C. *Governing Council 57. A Session of the Regional Committee*. Retrieved 12/31/2019, from https://www.paho.org/spanish/gov/cd/cd46-16-s.pdf?ua=1
PAHO/WHO. (2009). WHO case definition of HIV infection for surveillance purposes and revision of clinical staging and immunological classification of HIV-related disease in adults and children". Washington, D.C.: PAHO, 2009. ISBN: 978-9275-33279-5. Retrieved on 12/30/2019, from http://new.paho.org/hq/dmdocuments/2009/DEFINICION_ESTADIFICACION2.pdf
Ortiz, A., Estigarribia, G., Aguila, r. G., Espinosa Miranda, A., Mc Farland, W., Rfos-Gonzalez, C., ... Rodriguez, A. (2018). Prevalence of s^philis and behavioural characteristics of ind^genous youth in Paraguay, 2016. *Mem. Inst. Investig. Sci. Health., 16*(3), 5157 Doi: 10.18004/Mem.iics/1812-9528/2018.016(03)51-057. Retrieved 30 of 12
of 2019, of
https://revistascientificas.una.py/index.php/RIIC/article/view/1463/1410%2014/12/19
Osatnik, G., & Matsuya, C. (2013). The forced increase of the "Replenishment" resource generates risks due to loss of quality of the average haemodonant measured by HIV prevalence. *Rev. Arg. de Transf Vol XXXIX N°3, XXXIX* (3), 117. Retrieved on 12/31/2019, from https://www.aahitc.org.ar/rat/RAT032013.pdf
PAHO/ CHA HT/13.01 World Health Organization. (2013). HIV testing and counselling service delivery methods: a strategic programme framework. Washington, D.C. (PAHO, Ed.) ISBN 978-92-75-31778-5. Retrieved on 12/31/2019, from https://www.paho.org/hq/dmdocuments/2013/vih-metodos-provision-detection-2013.pdf
Patino Bedoya, J., Cortes Marquez, M., & Cardona Arias, J. (2012). Seroprevalence of markers of transfusion-transmissible infections in blood banks in Colombia. *Rev. Saude Publica, 46*(6), 950-9.

Retrieved on 12/31/2019, from http://www.scielo.br/pdf/rsp/v46n6/04.pdf
Paz, S., Adrover, R., & Ramadan, A. (November 2013). Session: Epidemiology and Prophylaxis. Lecture: i.Who should be screened for HCV? Advantages and disadvantages of universal screening. (AAEEH, Ed.) *Consenso Argentino de Hepatitis C. Book of abstracts*, pages 54-56.
PHAO/CHA/CD/Control de enfermedad de Chagas. (2014). *transmission by the main vector.* Retrieved on 15 01 01 2020, from https://www.paho.org/hq/dmdocuments/2014/Map-int-trans-vector-chagas.pdf
Piwowar-Manning, E., Fogel, J. R., Wolf, S., Clarke, W., Marzinke, M., Fiamma, A., ... Eshleman, S. (January 2015). Performance of the fourth-generation Bio-Rad GS HIV Combo Ag/Ab enzyme immunoassay for diagnosis of HIV infection in Southern Africa. *J Clin Virol., 62*, 75-79. doi:10.1016/j.jcv.2014.11.023. Retrieved on 12/31/2019, from https://jhu.pure.elsevier.com/en/publications/performance-of-the-fourth-generation- bio-rad-gs-hiv-combo-agab-en-3.
National Blood Donor Plan, Ministry of Health, (n.d.). *Criteria for blood donor selection*. Retrieved 15 01/01/2020, from http://iah.salud.gob.ar/doc/Documento117.pdf
Posada-Vergara, M., Montanheiro, P., Fukumori, L., Bonasser, F., Duarte, A. d., Penalva De Oliveira, A., & Casseb, J. (July-August 2006). Clinical and epidemiological aspects of HTLV-II infection in Sao Paulo, Brazil: presence of tropical spastic paraparesis/HTLVV- associated myelopathy (tsp/ham) simile diagnosis in hiv-1-co-infected subjects. *Rev. Inst. Med. trop. S. Paulo, 48*(4), 207-210. Retrieved on 12/31/2019, from http://www.scielo.br/pdf/rimtsp/v48n4/a06v48n4.pdf
Quesada Aramburu, J; Cadelli, E. (December 2012). Hacia una clasificacion de los municipios bonaerenses Documento de Trabajo DPEPE N°04/2012 Direccion Provincial de Estudios y Proyecciones Economicas, Min. de Econom^a, Pcia Bs As. Retrieved 12/31/2019, from https://observatoriosocial.unlam.edu.ar/descargas/6_Haciaunaclasificacindelosmunici piosbonaerenses.pdf
Rabinovich, R., Drakeley, C., Djimde, A., Fenton, H. B., Hay, S., Hemingway, J., ... Alonso, P. (30 November 2017). malERA: An updated research agenda for malaria elimination and eradication. *PLoS Med, 14*(11), e1002456 . https://doi.org/10.1371/journal.pmed.1002456. Retrieved on 12/31/2019, from https://journals.plos.org/plosmedicine/article?id=10.1371/journal.pmed.1002456
Ramos-Ligonio, A., Ramfrez-Sanchez, M., Gonzalez-Hernandez, J., Rosales-Encina, J., & Lopez-Monteon, A. (January-February 2006). Prevalence of antibodies against Trypanosoma cruzi in blood donors of IMSS, Orizaba, Veracruz, Mexico. *salud publica de Mexico/ vol.48, no.1,,, 48*(1). Retrieved 02 01/01/2020, from https://www.medigraphic.com/pdfs/salpubmex/sal-2006/sal061c.pdf
Raya, SM; Brunet, MM; Laura Norma Gomez, LN; Laperuta, VA; Parisi, NM; Rossini, JP; Brangold, M; Ponce, M; Bruzzone, M; (Aug 2017). *Plan de salud CABA 2016-2030. Ministry of Health, GCBA.* Retrieved 11 Jan 2020, from http://lista10.com.ar/site/wp-content/uploads/2017/11/Plan-del-Ministerio-de-Salud- 2030-digital.pdf
Real Delor, R., Moral, A., & Perez, L. (January - June 2016). Prevalence of human lymphotropic virus in Blood Donors of the National Hospital, Paraguay. *Rev. Med La Paz, 22*(1), 5-12. Retrieved on 12/31/2019, from http://www.scielo.org.bo/pdf/rmcmlp/v22n1/v22n1_a02.pdf
Recoder, ML; Nadal, M. (2016). *HIV diagnosis Recommendations for pre- and post-test counselling Edition 2016. Direction de Sida y ETS, Ministerio de Salud de la Nation. Argentina.* Retrieved on 12/31/2019, from http://www.msal.gob.ar/images/stories/bes/graficos/0000000117cnt-2016-12_guia- diagnostico-counseling.pdf
Reesink, H., Panzer, S., McQuilten, Z., Wood, E., Marks, D., Wendel, S., ... Castro, E. (July 2010). Pathogen inactivation of platelet concentrates. *Vox Sanguinis, 99*, 85-95 DOI: 10.1111/j.1423-0410.2010.01319.x. Retrieved on 12/31/2019, from

https://onlinelibrary.wiley.com/doi/abs/10.1111/j.1423-0410.2010.01319.x
Riveron Corteguera, R. (Jan-Mar 2002). Emerging and re-emerging diseases: a challenge for the 21st century. *Rev. Cubana Pediatr v.74 n.1 Ciudad de la Habana Jan-Mar. 2002 ISSN 1561-3119, 74*(1), ISSN 1561-3119. Retrieved on 12/31/2019, from http://scielo.sld.cu/scielo.php?pid=S0034-75312002000100002&script=sci_arttext&tlng=pt%2025/12/17
Rodrigues Coura, J. (May 2015). The main sceneries of Chagas disease transmission. The vectors, blood and oral transmissions - A comprehensive review. *Mem Inst Oswaldo Cruz, 110*(3), 277-282. Retrieved on December 31, 2019, from https://www.ncbi.nlm.nih.gov/pmc/articles/PMC4489464/pdf/0074-0276-mioc-110-3- 0277.pdf
Romany F. (2010). Systematic review of epidemiological studies on human T-cell lymphotropic virus I/II infection in Peru. *Rev. Peru. Epidemiol, 14*(3), 9 pp. ISSN-e 1609-7211. Retrieved on 01 01 2020, from https://dialnet.unirioja.es/servlet/articulo?codigo=3990188
Rossi, A., & Godoy, E. (2017). Loyalty of voluntary donors vs replacement donors. *Rev. Arg. de Transf., XLIII*(3), 198-199. Retrieved on January 08, 2020, from https://www.aahitc.org.ar/wp-content/uploads/2017/10/Revista-Argentina-de- Transfusi%C3%B3n-3-2017-.pdf
Rovira, C., Picagua, E. F., Gimenez, V., Carpinelli, M., & Granado, E. (June 2009). Prevalence of serological markers of viral hepatitis in a selected population.
Experience of a university service. Years 2000-2007. *Mem. Inst. Investig. Sci. Health,, 7*(1). Retrieved 01 01 2020, from http://scielo.iics.una.py/pdf/iics/v7n1/v7n1a04.pdf
San Miguel, C., Vera Cabral, E., & Fanego, H. (2010). Seroprevalence of S^filis in pregnant women in Alto Parana-2008. *Rev. Inst. Med. Trop., 5*(1), 7-13. Retrieved on 01 01 2020, from http://scielo.iics.una.py/pdf/imt/v5n1/v5n1a02.pdf
Sanchez Frenes, P., Sanchez Bouza, M. d., & Hernandez Malpica, S. (October - December 2012). Infectious diseases and blood transfusion. *Rev. Latinoamerican Patol Clin, 59*(4), 186-193. Retrieved on 01 01 2020, from https://www.medigraphic.com/pdfs/patol/pt-2012/pt124c.pdf
Sanodze, L., Bautista, C., Garuchava, N., Chubinidze, S., Tsertsvadze, E., Broladze, M., . . . Trapaidze, N. (2015). Expansion of brucellosis detection in the country of Georgia by screening household members of cases and neighboring community members. *BMC Public Health, 459*(15), DOI 10.1186/s12889-015-1761-y. Retrieved 01 01 2020, from https://bmcpublichealth.biomedcentral.com/articles/10.1186/s12889-015- 1761-y
Schmunis, G., & Cruz, J. (Jan 2005). Safety of the Blood Supply in Latin America. *Clinical Microbiology Reviews, 18*, 12-29 DOI: 10.1128/CMR.18.3.582.2005. Retrieved 01/01/202020, from https://cmr.asm.org/content/18/3/582
Schmunis, G. (1999). Risk of Chagas disease through transfusions in the Americas. *MEDICINA (Buenos Aires), 59*(Suppl. II), 125-134. Retrieved on 01 01 2020, from https://pdfs.semanticscholar.org/cb6c/8a11c6204edff87157a92c42ebc250db8407.pdf
Scialfa, E., Aguirre, P., & Bolpe, J. (n.d.). Characteristics of peri-urban family farms for food production and their relationship with prevalent zoonoses. Retrieved on 01 01 01 2020, from http://extension.unicen.edu.ar/jem/completas/57.pdf
Secretaria de Promocion y Programas Sanitarios, Ministerio de Salud, Argentina (January 2013). *Boletin Integrado de Vigilancia N° 156 SE 4.* Retrieved 12/23/2019, from https://www.argentina.gob.ar/sites/default/files/boletinintegradodevigilanciaversion_ n156-se4.pdf
Secretaria de Promocion y Programas Sanitarios, Ministry of Health, Argentina (February 2018). *Boletin Integrado de Vigilancia N° 397- SE 05 ISSN 2422-698X.* Retrieved on 12/23/2019, from https://www.argentina.gob.ar/sites/default/files/biv_397_se05- 2.pdf
Secretaria de Promocion y Programas Sanitarios, Ministerio de Salud, Argentina (January 2012). *Boletin Integrado de Vigilancia N° 106-SE 4.* Retrieved 12/23/2019, from

https://www.argentina.gob.ar/sites/default/files/boletinintegradodevigilanciaversion_ n106-se04.pdf

Secretaria de Promocion y Programas Sanitarios, Ministerio de Salud, Argentina (February 2014). *Boletin Integrado de Vigilancia N° 203 SE 3 Secretaria de Promocion y programas sanitarios MSAL Argentina.* Retrieved on December 23, 2019, from https://www.argentina.gob.ar/sites/default/files/biv-n203-se3.pdf

Serrano Machuca, J., Villarreal Rfos, E., Galicia Rodriguez, L., Vargas, D. E., Marrinez Gonzalez, L., & Mejia Damian, A. (2009). Detection of circulating antibodies in blood donors in Mexico. *Rev. Panam Salud Publica, 26*(4), 355-9. Retrieved on 01 01 2020, from https://www.scielosp.org/pdf/rpsp/2009.v26n4/355-359/es

Sguassero, Y., Cuesta, C., Roberts, K., Hicks, E., Comande, D., Ciapponi, A., & Sosa-Estani, S. (Oct 2015). Course of Chronic Trypanosoma cruzi Infection after Treatment Based on Parasitological and Serological Tests: A Systematic Review of Follow-Up Studies. *PLoS ONE, 10*(10), e0139363. Retrieved on 01 01 2020, from https://journals.plos.org/plosone/article?id=10.1371/journal.pone.0139363

Stienlauf, S., Yahalom, V., Schwartz, E., Shinar, E., Segal, G., & Sidi, Y. (July 2009). Epidemiology of Human T-cell Lymphotropic Virus Type 1 Infection in Blood Donors, Israel. *Emerging Infectious Diseases, 15*(7), DOI: 10.3201/eid1507.080796. Retrieved 02 01/01/2020, from https://wwwnc.cdc.gov/eid/article/15/7/pdfs/08-0796.pdf

Suarez Larreinaga, C., & Berdasquera Corcho, D. (2000). Emerging and re-emerging diseases: causal factors and surveillance. *Rev. Cubana Med Gen Integr, 16*(6), 5937. Retrieved 02 01/01/2020, from http://scielo.sld.cu/pdf/mgi/v16n6/mgi11600.pdf

Takatani, M., Crispim, M., Fraiji, N., Araujo, S. M., & Kiesslich, D. (2017). Clinical and laboratory features of HTLV-I asymptomatic carriers and patients with HTLV-I-associated myelopathy/ tropical spastic paraparesis from the Brazilian Amazon. *Rev Inst Med Trop Sao Paulo,* 59:e5. Retrieved 02 01/01/2020, from http://www.scielo.br/pdf/rimtsp/v59/1678-9946-rimtsp-59-e5.pdf

Thorstensson, R., Albert, J., & Andersson, S. (Jun 2002). Strategies for diagnosis of HTLV-I and -II. *Transfusion, 42*(6), 780-91. DOI: 10.1046/j.1537-2995.2002.00114.x. Retrieved 04 Jan 2020, from https://onlinelibrary.wiley.com/doi/epdf/10.1046/j.1537-2995.2002.00114.x?tracking_action=preview_click&r3_referer=wol&show_checkout= 1

Tillmann, H. (14 June 2014). Hepatitis C virus core antigen testing: Role in diagnosis, disease monitoring and treatment. *World J Gastroenterol 2014 June 14; 20(22): 67016706 DOI:10.3748/wjg.v20.i22.6701, 20*(22), 6701-6706 DOI:10.3748/wjg.v20.i22.6701. Retrieved 03 01 Jan 2020, from https://www.wjgnet.com/1007-9327/full/v20/i22/6701.htm

Truelove, S., & Hogben, L. (1947). Documentary study of jaundice associated with syphilis treatment and blood transfusion. *Brit. J. Soc. Med., 1,* 18-32. Retrieved 04 Jan 2020, from https://www.ncbi.nlm.nih.gov/pmc/articles/PMC1012498/pdf/brjsocmed00001- 0021.pdf

Tsegay, A., Tuli, G., Kassa, T., & Kebede, N. (2017). Seroprevalence and risk factors of brucellosis in abattoir workers at Debre Zeit and Modjo export abattoir, Central Ethiopia . *BMC Infectious Diseases,* 17:101 DOI 10.1186/s12879-017-2208-0. Retrieved 04 Jan 2020, from https://bmcinfectdis.biomedcentral.com/track/pdf/10.1186/s12879-017-2208-0?site=bmcinfectdis.biomedcentral.com

Varela, T; Fandino, ME; Baldiviezo, L; Ferro, N; Wainziger, T. (2019). *458° Boleti'n Integrado de Vigilancia Semana Epidemiologica 28/2019 Ministerio de Salud y Desarrollo Social de la Nation. Direction National de Epidemiologie et d'Analyse de la Situation de Santé ISSN 2422-698X {on line}.* Retrieved 05 01/01/2020, from https://www.argentina.gob.ar/sites/default/files/biv_458_se28_semanal2_1.pdf

Vladimirsky, S., Munne, M., Otegui, L., Altabert, N., Soto, S., & Brajterman, L. (2015). Sentinel Units for viral hepatitis, Gonzalez JE Registry of patients with hepatitis C in the Sentinel Units for viral hepatitis in Argentina, 2007 -2014. Distribution by year of birth. *Acta Gastroenterol Latinoam, 45*(2), 110-116. Retrieved 05 01/05/202020, from http://www.actagastro.org/numeros-anteriores/2015/Vol-45- N2/Vol45N2-PDF07.pdf

Vladimirsky, S., Munne, M., Otegui, L., Altabert, N., Soto, S., Brajterman, L., ... Gonzalez, J. (2013). Viral hepatitis surveillance in Argentina: Analysis of information obtained by Sentinel Units 2007-2010. *Acta Gastroenterol Latinoam, 43*(1), 22-30. Retrieved 05 01/01/202020, from http://www.actagastro.org/numeros- anteriores/2013/Vol-43-N1/Vol43N1-PDF10.pdf.

Webster, D., Klenerman, P., & Dusheiko, G. (March 21, 2015). Hepatitis C. *The Lancet, 385*(9973), 1124-1135. Retrieved 05 01 Jan 2020, from https://www.thelancet.com/action/showPdf?pii=S0140-6736%2814%2962401-6

Welch, N., Easton, C., Scoble, J., Williams, C., Pigram, P., & Muir, B. (2016). A chemiluminescent sandwich ELISA enhancement method using a chromium (III) coordination complex. *Journal of Immunological Methods, 438*, 59-66. Retrieved on 05 01, 2020, from https://www.sciencedirect.com/science/article/abs/pii/S0022175916301995?via%3Di hub

WHO (2017). Global Hepatitis Report 2017. Geneva: World Health Organization. ISBN 978-924-156545-5 . Retrieved 05 01 Jan 2020, from https://apps.who.int/iris/bitstream/handle/10665/255016/9789241565455- eng.pdf?sequence=1

WHO (n.d.). *Global and Country Estimates of immunization coverage and chronic HBV infection.* Retrieved 15 Jan. 01, 2020, from http://whohbsagdashboard.com/#global- strategies.

WHO/HSE/PED/HIP/GHP. (2012). *Prevention and control of viral hepatitis: Framework for global action World Health Organization 2012.* Retrieved 05 Jan. 01, 2020, from https://apps.who.int/iris/bitstream/handle/10665/130014/WHO_HSE_PED_HIP_GHP_ 2012.1_spa.pdf;jsessionid=8D8F80FFE3CCE0C3FEE0AE385BCE64CE?sequence=1

Wick, M., Moore, S., & Taswell, H. (Mar-Apr 1895). Non-A, non-B hepatitis associated with blood transfusion. *Transfusion , 25*(2), 93-101. Retrieved 05 01/05/2020, from https://onlinelibrary.wiley.com/doi/pdf/10.1046/j.1537-2995.1985.25285169225.x

Wood, E. (1 Jan 1955). Brucellosis as a hazard of blood transfusion. *Br Med J. , 1(4904),* 27-8 DOI: 10.1136/bmj.1.4904.27. Retrieved 05 01/01/2020, from https://www.ncbi.nlm.nih.gov/pmc/articles/PMC2060716/pdf/brmedj03319-0033.pdf

Zambrano Plata, G., & Cortez, J. (2001) Seroprevalence of HIV, Hepatitis B Hepatitis C, Chagas and S^filis in blood bank donors in Cucuta (Colombia) 1998-1999. *Respuestas, 6*(1), 45-49 , ISSN 0122-820X, ISSN-e 2422-5053,. Retrieved 05 01/01/202020, from https://dialnet.unirioja.es/servlet/articulo?codigo=5555289

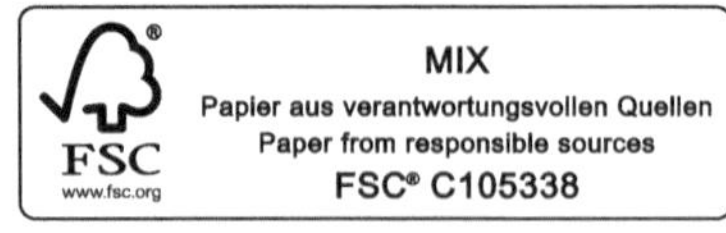

Printed by Books on Demand GmbH, Norderstedt / Germany